Epidemiology of Hospital-Associated Infections

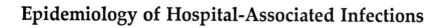

Epidemiology of Hospital-Associated Infections

Peter C. Fuchs, M.D., Ph.D.

Hospital Epidemiologist
Department of Pathology
St. Vincent Hospital and Medical Center
Portland, Oregon

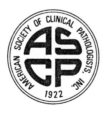

Educational Products Division
American Society of Clinical Pathologists
Chicago

Library of Congress Cataloging in Publication Data

Fuchs, Peter C.
    Epidemiology of hospital-associated infections.

    Bibliography: **p.**
    Includes index.
    1. Nosocomial infections. 2. Epidemiology.
I. Title.
RC112.F8   614.4   79-17036
ISBN 0-89189-072-6

Contents

Contents

Preface

The past ten to fifteen years have witnessed the initiation and rapid proliferation of hospital epidemiology programs throughout the country—despite the absence of concrete documentation of their effectiveness. This is undoubtedly due in part to the fact that such programs are now required by hospital accrediting agencies. On the other hand, there is considerable circumstantial evidence that properly functioning epidemiology programs play an important role in keeping nosocomial infection rates as low as modern knowledge and technology permit.

The aims of this treatise are threefold: (1) to provide an overall picture of the problem of nosocomial infections as it exists in health care institutions today; (2) to provide basic information relative to the epidemiology of nosocomial infections with emphasis on underlying and predisposing factors, types of infections that occur, and the more important etiologic agents; and (3) to provide a guide for conducting a hospital epidemiology program, including defining the roles of the epidemiologist and other personnel in the control of nosocomial infections.

To fulfill these goals adequately would require lengthening this manuscript severalfold. In order to avoid this, a compromise was made by which many topics are discussed somewhat superficially but are appended by a liberal number of references for those wishing to pursue them in greater detail. In addition to the specific cited references, there is a list of general references at the end that cover various aspects of hospital epidemiology.

I am deeply indebted to the following individuals for their help and advice in the preparation of this manuscript: Marie Gustafson, Louise Jones, Ronald N. Jones, Carol Pelton, and Stephen Stolzberg. I also wish to thank my wife and children for their understanding and indulgence.

PETER C. FUCHS

Chapter 1:
Introduction

HISTORY

Nosocomial infections (infections acquired by patients in health care institutions) have a history coexistent with that of health care institutions. The common expectation is that persons admitted to hospitals should recover from illnesses, not acquire them. In fact, however, infection risks in health care institutions may be higher than those in the community. Among the many reasons contributing to this are the following:

1. Health care facilities are not totally isolated from the community and therefore are subject to most of the same infection risks (endemic and epidemic).
2. Persons with serious infections are frequently admitted to hospitals and thus provide an intrahospital reservoir of pathogenic microbes.
3. The proportion of people with increased susceptibility to infections is much greater in the hospital population than in the community at large.

Prior to the germ theory, putrefaction and contagious illnesses in hospitals were generally accepted as inevitable. The underlying mechanisms and epidemiology were unknown. Aside from isolation of patients tantamount to abandonment, no means of breaking the chain of contagion was established before the mid-19th century. Physicians such as Oliver Wendell Holmes and Ignaz Philip Semmelweis suggested and demonstrated the effectiveness of hand-washing in reducing the incidence of puerperal sepsis in hospitals. A contemporary, Joseph Lister, demonstrated in 1865 the efficacy of using carbolic acid as an antiseptic in the prevention of surgical wound infections. Both of these milestones (hand-washing and surgical asepsis) remain even today as the most basic principles in the prophylaxis of nosocomial infections.

The work of Louis Pasteur, Robert Koch, and many others increased our understanding of the microbial cause of infection, from which emerged such concepts as virulence, inoculum size, and portal of entry. The idea of host factors also had its beginning in the work of Pasteur and his vaccines for anthrax and rabies. The concept emerged that persons develop immunity to an infectious agent following previous exposure to the agent. Cellular immune mechanisms were first reported by Elie Metchnikoff in the late 19th century. Over the following decades the concepts of cellular and humoral immunity made slow progress, but during the past 20 to 30 years the advances have been gigantic and rapid. It is beyond the scope of this text to delve into these, but the interested reader may wish to review modern standard treatises.

In recent years the concept of the *compromised host* has emerged as a significant factor in nosocomial infections. This refers to any host in whom any defense mechanism against infection is weakened or deficient. In the broad sense, the vast majority of hospitalized patients are compromised hosts. Even the immunocompetent patient admitted for elective surgery becomes a compromised host at the time of surgery when a major defense barrier against infection—the skin—is incised. More commonly, however, the term is used in a restricted sense to denote hosts who are immunologically (humoral or cellular immunity) compromised.

The compromised immunologic state of many patients today is iatrogenic. It is true that congenital immunologic deficiencies occur and such hosts are highly susceptible to infections, but these are relatively rare. Some diseases are associated with impaired immune mechanisms, but in the past most patients with such diseases died before infections associated with the compromised immune state occurred. Modern medical therapy has altered this pattern by at least two mechanisms. First, the increased life-span of patients who have illnesses that are secondarily associated with immune deficiencies (eg, leukemia, lymphoma, other malignancies, and diabetes mellitus) has provided greater opportunity for the development and manifestation of these immunologic defects. Second, a major undesired secondary effect of many of the therapeutic modalities themselves has been significant immunosuppression (eg, x-irradiation, corticosteroids, and antineoplastic drugs). Frequently the two mechanisms operate simultaneously in the same patient. This has resulted not only in an increased infection rate but also in serious and often fatal infections by microbes that were formerly considered nonpathogenic and often constitute part of the normal host flora. Such pathogens that are generally unable to produce infection in a competent host but do produce infections in a compromised host are referred to as *opportunistic pathogens*. Most normal microbial flora are capable of being opportunistic pathogens under appropriate circumstances.

Local defense mechanisms frequently are compromised by both diagnostic and therapeutic modalities. Although the mechanisms are not entirely clear, it is well recognized that foreign bodies locally reduce resistance to infection. The insertion of foreign devices is common in medical practice today (eg, indwelling urinary and intravascular catheters, pacemakers, prosthetic joints, heart valves, and vessels). The sites of such implants exhibit increased susceptibility to infection whether microbes are introduced at the time of implantation or the sites are subsequently seeded by bacteremic episodes.

Antimicrobial chemotherapy also has had some undesirable side effects. Although the introduction of antibiotics has been the most significant advance in medical history from the standpoint of reduction of morbidity and mortality, the microbe world has not accepted this assault without retaliation. Many microbes have developed means of resistance to each new antimicrobic as it becomes available. Consequently, the use of therapeutic and prophylactic antimicrobics has resulted not only in cures and fewer infections, respectively, but also in colonization and infection of the host by antibiotic-resistant microbes, which are often very difficult to eradicate.

Thus, over the years progress in medicine has brought about a change in the pattern of nosocomial infections from one of primary pathogenic microbes in relatively immunocompetent hosts to that of opportunistic drug-resistant pathogens in compromised hosts. Whereas the former pattern was accepted as inevitable and nonpreventable prior to the 19th century, methods of controlling this pattern are now well established. Today there is a tendency to accept the current pattern of opportunistic infections in compromised hosts as inevitable and nonpreventable. Our obvious challenge is to find the means to control this new pattern of nosocomial infections.

INFECTIONS

DEFINITIONS

A dissertation on nosocomial infections must be based on a precise concept of infection. Many terms describe various relationships between microbes and hosts. Brief definitions of such terms used in this text follow:

Carrier state.—The state of persistent colonization or asymptomatic infection of a host by a specific microbial species—usually one with significant pathogenic potential, eg, Staphylococcus aureus, Salmonella species, hepatitis B virus.

Colonization.—The populating of body areas (eg, skin or mucous membranes) by microbes, with no tissue invasion or production of clinical disease.

Commensalism.—The association between a host and microbe that results in neither benefit nor harm to either.

Contamination.—The transient undesired occurrence of microbes on animate or inanimate surfaces.

Endogenous infection.—Infection caused by microbes derived from the host's own flora.

Exogenous infection.—Infection caused by microbes derived from outside the host.

Flora.—The normal microbial population and other colonizers of body surfaces.

Immune state.—A host state of relative resistance to invasion (and colonization?) by specific microbes.

Infection.—The invasion of host tissue by one or more microbial species usually detrimental to the host, with the resulting production of clinical disease.

Symbiosis.—The association between a host and microbe that is mutually advantageous.

All of the above are common relationships between hosts and the microbial world. Only infection is clearly deleterious to the host. In practice, these relationships are not always so black and white as suggested by these definitions. Shades of gray are common, particularly in the setting of a health care facility. Infections are usually recognized by signs and symptoms that are manifestations of the host's response to this microbial invasion. In hospitals many patients are elderly, debilitated, or immunosuppressed by disease or therapy and, hence, are unable to respond to infection in the usual manner—if at all. In such patients the recognition of infection or the differentiation of infection from colonization may be extremely difficult.

CRITERIA

Although the definition of infection given above may evoke no major objections, the criteria by which particular host-microbe relationships are recognized or identified as infections are often controversial. This is often the case, for example, in distinguishing between infection and colonization of the urinary tract, respiratory tract, and even wounds. Consequently, for assessment purposes it is important to establish a set of criteria whereby particular cases can be determined to be infections or not infections. Although the accuracy of such criteria is highly desirable, it is perhaps more important that the criteria ensure consistency in making such distinctions. It is only in this way that one can assess infection rates and problems in an institution over a period of time, or compare infections in one institution with those in another. The criteria listed in Table 1-1 for the identification of various types of infection are those utilized by the Hospital Infections Section of the Center for Disease Control (CDC).[116] These criteria will not be acceptable to everyone, but for those who can work with them, they will provide a basis of comparison with many other institutions.

Four factors interact in determining whether or not an infection will occur: the size of the microbial inoculum, the virulence of the microbe, the portal of entry, and the immune status of the host. Each of these factors is intimately related to and dependent on the others. The size of the microbial inoculum required to initiate an infection is inversely related to the virulence of the organism, is directly related to the immune status of the host, and depends variably on the portal of entry provided. Prior to the modern era of medicine, the microbial factors (ie, virulence and inoculum size) were considered the major determinants in infection. Today, host factors play an increasingly important role.

TABLE 1-1.—Criteria for Infections at Specific Sites

I. Urinary tract infections
    A. Colony counts greater than 10^5 colony-forming units (CFU)/ml with or without symptoms
    B. Urinary tract infection symptoms (fever, dysuria, costovertebral angle (CVA) tenderness, etc) with one or more of the following
        1. Colony counts greater than 10^4 CFU/ml
        2. Microbes visible in unspun urine smear
        3. Pyuria with more than 10 WBC/high-power field (HPF) in unspun urine

II. Respiratory tract infections
    A. Signs and symptoms of upper respiratory tract infection with or without positive microbe culture
    B. Signs and symptoms of lower respiratory tract infection with one or more of the following
        1. Purulent sputum
        2. Pathogen recovered from sputum or blood
        3. Suggestive chest x-ray

III. Skin and subcutaneous infections
    A. Surgical wounds, traumatic wounds, ulcers, and other lesions that drain purulent material—with or without positive microbe cultures
    B. Cellulitis
    C. Burns with purulent drainage and/or bacteremia
    D. Surgical wounds of infected regions that become infected are *not* considered separate infections

IV. Gastroenteritis
    A. Symptomatic gastroenteritis associated with culture positive for an enteric pathogen

TABLE 1-1.—Criteria for Infections at Specific Sites *(cont.)*

    B. Symptomatic gastroenteritis with strong epidemiologic evidence of infectious etiology

V. Miscellaneous
    A. Bacteremia with or without a known source
    B. Intravascular implement infection
       1. Purulent drainage from site
       2. Inflammation or cellulitis with positive culture
    C. Endometritis—purulent cervical drainage with one or more of the following
       1. Positive culture of pathogen
       2. Systemic signs and symptoms of infection
    D. Intra-abdominal infections
       1. Abscess, peritonitis
       2. *Not* uncomplicated appendicitis, diverticulitis, cholecystitis
    E. Other sites—signs and symptoms of infection and/or positive pathogen cultures or serology

VI. Clinical diagnosis of infection at any site

NOSOCOMIAL INFECTIONS

The terms *hospital-acquired infections*, *hospital-associated infections*, and *nosocomial infections* are used interchangeably to designate an infection contracted by a person while hospitalized. The first two terms often imply hospital responsibility or culpability. Many infections that occur in hospitalized patients would have occurred in any event, but merely because the patients happen to be in a hospital, the infections are labeled "hospital-acquired." On the other hand, infections do develop in hospitalized persons that can be traced directly or indirectly to factors within the hospital, and these probably would not have occurred under other circumstances. Such infections are truly hospital-acquired or hospital-associated. The term *nosocomial infection*, at least at the present time, is free of the connotation of hospital culpability and includes both types of infections depicted above. This is the term that will be used here.

All infections that are not nosocomial by definition must have been acquired outside the hospital; they are community-acquired infections. Determining whether an infection is nosocomial or community-acquired is occasionally much more difficult in practice than in theory. The difficulty arises from the variable lengths of incubation periods of different infections. If all infections became clinically manifest at the moment they were acquired, there would be no problem in classifying them. In fact, however, infections become clinically manifest in hospitalized patients who are admitted while in the incubation period of community-acquired infections, and nosocomial infections may become clinically manifest sometime after the patient is discharged from the hospital. Furthermore, the incubation periods of many infections are too imprecise and variable to be useful as a sole criterion to determine retrospectively the moment of acquisition of an infection.

It therefore becomes necessary to set up reasonable criteria for categorizing infections that are not of patent nosocomial or community origin. If one wishes to record infection rates within an institution over a period of time or to compare infection statistics with those of other institutions, it is essential that the criteria permit consistent classification. For our purposes the criteria established by the Hospital Infections Section of the Center for Disease Control (CDC) will be used.[116] These are summarized in Table 1-2. Although a number of these criteria may be controversial, they do provide a means of comparing the statistics of a large number of institutions that currently use them. If, however, an institution and its medical staff are unable to accept these criteria, the statistical data will be far more meaningful if that institution establishes its own criteria that are acceptable and implementable than if it attempts to enforce the CDC criteria.

TABLE 1-2.—Criteria for Categorizing Infections as Nosocomial

---

I. Infections not present or incubating at time of admission

II. Infections present on admission but acquired from a previous admission

III. Infections manifest after discharge but acquired during hospitalization

IV. Appearance of new organism in previous infection site—if clinical manifestations persist or worsen

V. Infection at a new site by the same organism, causing infection at a separate site

VI. Generalizations regarding common specific site infections

    A. Postoperative wound infections—if not secondary to surgery in an infected field

    B. Urinary tract infections

       1. After instrumentation

       2. After catheterization

TABLE 1-2.—Criteria for Categorizing Infections as Nosocomial *(cont.)*

---

 3. Occurring after 48 hours if admission urine test results were normal
C. Respiratory tract infections
 1. After anesthesia
 2. After respiratory therapy
 3. Occurring after 48 hours if patient was asymptomatic on admission
D. Intravascular implement site infections

In recent years it has been recognized that persons admitted to health care facilities become colonized by microbes indigenous to the institution. The prevalence of such colonization correlates with the length of hospitalization[548] and the clinical severity of illness.[299] Nosocomial endogenous infections that develop in such persons may be caused by either hospital-acquired microbes or community-acquired microbes. The epidemiologic classification of infections seen in health care institutions is given in Table 1-3.

TABLE 1-3.—Classification of Hospital Infections

 I. Community-acquired infections
 II. Nosocomial infections
  A. Exogenous infections
  B. Endogenous infections
   1. Community microbes
   2. Hospital microbes

This classification obviously is an oversimplification of complex interactions. One could also make a case for considering infections by hospital microbes following colonization as exogenous infections. Certainly the ultimate source of such microbes is the hospital (exogenous), but at the time the infection occurs, the source is the patient's flora (endogenous). This then raises questions regarding the distinction between colonization and infection, the duration of colonization prior to infection, the mechanism of colonization, and others. The answers to most such questions remain largely speculative. There is evidence to indicate that major sources of colonization are food and hospital personnel.

The colonization of hospitalized patients by hospital microbes undoubtedly is an important factor in many nosocomial infections. The normal relationship between a host and the microbial flora of that host is one of mutual benefit and delicate balance. The microbial flora are provided a place of residence, while the host has developed a resistance or immune status against these organisms sufficient to prevent tissue invasion (infection) but without eliminating the carrier status. The microbial flora may benefit the host by producing an inhospitable environment for more pathogenic microbes—either by their physical presence or by the production of bacteriocins or other antimicrobial substances. Under the appropriate conditions, however, most of these normal microbial flora may become opportunistic pathogens. Staphylococci, for example, are part of the normal flora of the skin and are usually harmless. But if sufficient numbers are allowed to penetrate the skin barrier by some "abnormal" portal such as an intravenous cannula or surgical incision, infection may result. If, on the other hand, the person had become colonized by hospital staphylococci prior to the break in cutaneous integrity, the odds theoretically would favor infection. Time is required for the host to establish an optimal immune status against new microbial flora. If the conditions predisposing to development of infection occur shortly after colonization by an organism unfamiliar to the host, the host's resistance to infection by such an organism is weaker than that to one with which a commensal relationship already has been developed. Based on this, the following conclusions can be drawn: (1) With all other factors equal, a recent hospital-acquired colonizer is more apt to produce an infection than are established flora. (2) A smaller inoculum of recently acquired hospital microbial flora of equal pathogenicity is required to initiate an infection. (3) Less impairment of host resistance is required to permit infection by recently acquired hospital flora than by established normal flora of equal pathogenicity.

One final type of infection must be mentioned briefly because of controversy concerning its nosocomial status; that is, reactivated or recrudescent infections. Patients may harbor pathogenic microbes in a latent state, presumably held in check by host defenses; but when these deferses are diminished due to underlying diseases and/or immunosuppressive therapy, these pathogenic agents may be reactivated and produce clinical disease that may be severe and even fatal. Such agents may be viral, bacterial, protozoal, or metazoal. Despite the fact that the primary infections usually are community-acquired, it is our contention that the reactivation or recrudescence of those infections in the hospital setting justifies regarding them as nosocomial. Examples of such infections are listed in Table 1-4.

IMPACT OF NOSOCOMIAL INFECTIONS

It is generally stated that one patient in every 20 admitted to a hospital in the United States today will develop an infection he or she did not have on admission. This may vary considerably among different types of hospitals, but hospital size alone is not a significant determinant of the frequency of nosocomial infection.[74] Based on studies conducted by CDC, the nosocomial infection rate in the United States is estimated to be approximately 5.5%, or two million patients per year.[151] When one considers the morbidity, increased length of hospital stay, and mortality secondary to such infections, the magnitude of the problem becomes staggering. Based on estimations of excess days of hospitalization resulting from nosocomial infections, it has been calculated that the current direct cost of such infections is more than $1 billion annually.[56, 151, 537] In one retrospective study, patients with nosocomial bacteremias were hospitalized an average of 14 days longer than matched controls.[581] However, attempts to determine the amount of excess hospitalization due solely to nosocomial infections are fraught with difficulties. Many patients who develop nosocomial infections also have other complications that contribute to prolonged hospital stay. Furthermore, patients with longer-than-average hospital stays are sicker, have other complications, and hence are more likely to develop nosocomial infections the longer they remain in the hospital. Consequently, an analysis of the contribution of nosocomial infections to increased hospital stay becomes circuitous, and the figures obtained are little more than estimates or subjective judgments. In any event, there is little doubt that nosocomial infections do prolong hospital stay and are an economic liability. Although hospital infection control programs can be justified on many grounds, it would be appropriate if, in this era of cost containment, they could be justified on economic ones. If it could be shown that such programs reduce the nosocomial infection rate by as little as 0.5% (eg, from 5.5% to 5.0%), the economic savings would amply justify the modest cost of such programs. To date we are unaware of any study reporting such effectiveness. It has been estimated in one recent study, however, that the current direct costs of nosocomial infection are approximately 25% less than they would be if the infection control practices currently in use were discontinued.[56]

TABLE 1-4.—Examples of Reactivated Infections, Proven or Strongly
Suspected, Considered Nosocomial in a Hospital Setting

INFECTION	REFERENCES
Cytomegalovirus infection	193, 273, 404, 428, 496, 596
Epstein-Barr virus infection	117, 428, 592
Herpes simplex virus infection	412, 418, 428, 461, 497, 519
Histoplasma capsulatum	150
Measles	9
Mycobacterium tuberculosis	311
Plasmodium infection (malaria)	134
Pneumocystis carinii pneumonitis	472
Pseudomonas pseudomallei (melioidosis)	515
Strongyloides stercoralis (strongyloidiasis)	137, 175, 432, 509
Toxoplasma gondii (toxoplasmosis)	93, 128, 232, 527, 627
Varicella zoster (herpes zoster)	186, 233, 499, 538, 663

Chapter 2:
Mechanisms and Conditions
of Nosocomial Infections—
General Aspects

The identification of factors that predispose to nosocomial infections and the development of preventive and remedial measures constitute one of the primary thrusts of a hospital epidemiology program. Although many such factors remain to be discovered and elucidated, some are well known and recognized to be significant in nosocomial infections. Factors that are involved in the development of nosocomial infections can be grouped broadly as follows: (1) host factors, (2) portals of entry, (3) microbial factors, and (4) infection sites.

HOST FACTORS

A major condition of predisposition to nosocomial infection is the primary illness for which a patient is admitted to the hospital, eg, diabetes, malignancies, collagen-vascular diseases, traumatic injuries, or burns. The specific illness often predisposes to particular infections. Table 2–1 lists some examples of primary illnesses that are associated with unusual susceptibility to certain microbial infections.

A more significant host factor that predisposes to nosocomial infection is the immunosuppressed state that results in patients undergoing therapeutic measures commonly used in hospitals. These include, but are not limited to, corticosteroids, cytotoxic drugs, immunosuppressive drugs, radiation therapy, and previous splenectomy. Such therapeutic modalities not only may suppress cellular and/or humoral resistance mechanisms but also may be myelotoxic, resulting in profound neutropenia. Such states render patients more susceptible to infections by less virulent organisms from the environment as well as from their own microbial flora. Many of these therapeutic modalities are used in treating the conditions listed in Table 2–1. In addition, recrudescent infections are more likely to occur. Microbial infections from which the patient has recovered may persist in a latent form, held inactive by the patient's immune system; but when the immune system is suppressed, etiologic agents of such infections can be reactivated and produce severe disease (see Table 1-4).

A significant loss of resistance to infection occurs locally at the site of foreign bodies in the host. Foreign material is commonly implanted or inserted into patients for therapeutic reasons, eg, prosthetic heart valves, orthopedic hardware, urinary and intravenous catheters, or vascular grafts. Animal studies show well that the presence of a foreign body reduces the number of organisms needed to produce an infection at a particular site (James and MacLeod, 1961).

Age is also a major host factor. Immune mechanisms are immature in the newborn and deteriorate in the elderly. Consequently, neonates and the very old are more susceptible to infections, and this is manifested by higher infection rates in these groups (see Table 2-1).

In contrast to some of the items to be discussed later, little can be done to control these host factors. They are inherent in the patient's physiologic or pathologic state or in the therapy being administered. Vaccines soon may play a role in preventing infections in conditions of increased susceptibility to a limited number of specific microbes, eg, pneumococcal vaccines for patients with sickle cell anemia and splenectomized patients.[19] For the most part, however, infection in such patients currently must be controlled through treatment of microbial factors. Depending on the specific circumstances, measures such as protective isolation of these patients and the use of prophylactic antibiotics have been found to be variably successful in reducing infection rates in compromised hosts.

PORTALS OF ENTRY AND MECHANISMS OF TRANSMISSION

The skin and mucous membranes of body surfaces are effective mechanical barriers to the invasion of deeper tissue by microbes. Such body surfaces are normally heavily colonized by microbes that live in a commensal relationship with the host. There is evidence that the normal microbial flora may play an important role in protecting the host from colonization and infections by pathogenic microbes—both by their physical presence and by the elaboration of antimicrobial substances specific for certain pathogens. Whenever the intactness of the skin or mucosa is interrupted or disturbed significantly, the mechanical barrier function is weakened or lost, thus permitting entrance by both flora and environmental microbes. There are many therapeutic devices that permit microbial access to normally sterile parts of the body either by providing an easy portal of entry or by becoming contaminated and carrying the microbes directly to the susceptible area. Specific mechanisms of acquiring and transmitting nosocomial infections are discussed in subsequent chapters.

TABLE 2-1.—Examples of Underlying Conditions Associated with
Susceptibilities to Specific Microbes and Infections

UNDERLYING CONDITION	PATHOGEN	INFECTION*	REFERENCES
Burns	Aspergillus species	Burn wound	429
	Herpes simplex virus	Burn/systemic	199
	Phycomycetes	Burn wound	200, 429
	Providencia stuartii	Burn wound	325, 451
	Pseudomonas aeruginosa	Burn wound	334, 363, 668
Cystic fibrosis	Pseudomonas aeruginosa	Pulmonary	339, 661, 668
Diabetes mellitus	Bacteroides fragilis	Sepsis	71, 188
	Candida species	Sepsis	165, 442
	Phycomycetes	Miscellaneous	398
	Staphylococcus aureus	Miscellaneous	127, 569
	Streptococcus agalactiae	Sepsis	45, 356
	Torulopsis glabrata	Renal/miscellaneous	322, 454
Malignancies			
General	Aspergillus species	Pulmonary	399, 671
	Bacteroides fragilis	Sepsis	71, 188, 306
	Bacille Calmette Guérin	Hepatitis/systemic	286, 459, 508, 521, 523
	Candida species	Miscellaneous	144, 165, 173, 386, 421
	Clostridium septicum	Sepsis	12, 355
	Hepatitis B virus	Hepatitis	594, 635
	Herpes simplex virus	Miscellaneous	418, 519
	Listeria monocytogenes	Miscellaneous	217, 372
	Pseudomonas aeruginosa	Pulmonary/sepsis	196, 198, 471, 668
	Torulopsis glabrata	Miscellaneous	384
Lymphoma/leukemia	Aeromonas hydrophila	Sepsis	3, 229, 371, 465
(highest)	Cytomegalovirus	Systemic	273
	Phycomycetes	Miscellaneous	398, 458
	Pneumocystis carinii	Pulmonary	472, 555, 634
	Staphylococcus aureus	Miscellaneous	127, 478
	Strongyloides stercoralis	GI/systemic	509, 514
	Toxoplasma gondii	CNS/systemic	93, 232, 527, 627
Hodgkin's disease	Varicella zoster	Skin/systemic	186, 233, 499, 538, 663
Neonatal state	Chlamydia trachomatis	Eye/pulmonary	53, 210, 244, 266
	Citrobacter diversus	Meningitis	251, 257, 504
	Escherichia coli	Meningitis/diarrhea	391, 511, 528, 532, 624
	Flavobacterium meningosepticum	Meningitis	267, 380, 479
	Listeria monocytogenes	Meningitis/sepsis	10, 449
	Neisseria gonorrhoeae	Ophthalmia neonatorum	608
	Pseudomonas aeruginosa	Miscellaneous	69, 159, 194, 416
	Staphylococcus aureus	Miscellaneous	174, 202, 426
	Streptococcus agalactiae	Meningitis/sepsis	36, 460, 491
Organ transplant	Aspergillus species	Systemic	255, 533
	Cytomegalovirus	Systemic	193, 273, 404, 428, 437, 596
	Epstein-Barr virus	Systemic	117, 428, 592
	Herpes simplex virus	Miscellaneous	157, 412, 428, 497
	Nocardia asteroides	Systemic	30, 337, 474
	Pneumocystis carinii	Pulmonary	506
	Strongyloides stercoralis	GI/systemic	175
	Toxoplasma gondii	Systemic	128, 232, 502, 527
Paraplegia	Proteus rettgeri	UTI	290
	Providencia stuartii	UTI	575
Postpartum state	Streptococcus agalactiae	CNS/sepsis	353, 356
	Streptococcus pyogenes	Puerperal sepsis	298
Sickle cell anemia	Streptococcus pneumoniae	RTI/CNS/sepsis	546
Splenectomy	Streptococcus pneumoniae	Sepsis	66, 236

*Abbreviations: GI, gastrointestinal; CNS, central nervous system; UTI, urinary tract infection; RTI, respiratory tract infection.

MICROBIAL FACTORS

The two major microbial determinants of infection in general, ie, microbial virulence and inoculum size, are equally applicable to nosocomial infections and need not be discussed further here. There is, however, a third factor that is almost unique to the hospital setting—the prevalence of microbes that are resistant to many antimicrobial agents. The problem of drug-resistant microbes and their epidemiology, which is complex and multifaceted, has been discussed elsewhere.[195, 343] Only a few specific and pertinent aspects will be mentioned briefly.

ANTIMICROBIC RESISTANCE

Chromosomally mediated antimicrobic resistance.—Antimicrobic resistance in microbes may be either chromosomally or episomally (plasmid, R factor) mediated. Chromosomally mediated antimicrobic resistance may be an inherent characteristic of a particular species, eg, the resistance of *Proteus mirabilis* to tetracyclines and polymyxins. Or, resistant mutants may occur at determinable frequencies that emerge under the selective pressure of the appropriate antimicrobic, eg, the resistance of *Mycobacterium tuberculosis* to streptomycin. In the absence of antimicrobics, resistant mutants that develop spontaneously enjoy no selective advantage over the prevalent susceptible microbes and will not emerge as problem organisms. This has some relevance epidemiologically because the prevalence of specific antimicrobic resistance among microbes in the hospital setting is often directly related to the use of the specific antimicrobic. A number of reports document the termination of nosocomial outbreaks caused by specific drug-resistant organisms after the antimicrobics to which the organisms were resistant are no longer used.[486] This is also one of the cogent arguments against the indiscriminate use of antimicrobics.

Plasmid-mediated antimicrobic resistance.—Plasmids are extrachromosomal, DNA-containing organelles of microorganisms; they not only replicate in normal cell division but also may be transferred (by transformation and, possibly, by transduction) to other members of the same or related species or may be lost spontaneously. Plasmids that mediate resistance to antimicrobics have been referred to as R factors or resistance plasmids. Examples of plasmid-mediated antimicrobic resistance include ampicillin-resistant *Hemophilus influenzae*, penicillinase-producing *Neisseria gonorrhoeae*, and chloramphenicol-resistant *Salmonella* species. There is a great diversity of R factors among the Enterobacteriaceae. Despite the theoretical potential problems that plasmid-mediated antimicrobic resistance could cause in the hospital setting, there is little evidence that such problems do in fact occur. Nevertheless, this is an area requiring much more study.

Prophylactic antimicrobial resistance. — Antimicrobial agents are used primarily in the treatment of infectious diseases, but increasingly they also are used in the prophylaxis of infections. Regardless of the purpose, one of the side effects of the use of systemic antimicrobics is an alteration of the microbial floral balance in favor of microbes that are resistant to the antimicrobic being used. When the appropriate conditions for infections or suprainfections prevail, the likelihood is enhanced that the infecting agent will be a resistant organism. In our experience, the use of prophylactic antimicrobics for various surgical procedures such as bowel resection has resulted in a definitely lower postoperative wound infection rate, but the infections that do occur often are due to more resistant organisms. Hence, the lowered infection rate does not come without a price.

INFECTION SITES

Urinary tract infections, respiratory tract infections, and postoperative wound infections account for more than 75% of the nosocomial infections reported in most studies. Most such studies, however, include primarily, if not exclusively, bacterial and fungal infections. The full spectrum and significance of nosocomial viral infection are not yet appreciated. In the subsequent chapters, there is a brief discussion of nosocomial infection in relation to the site of infection, including viral, bacterial, fungal, and parasitic infections.

Chapter 3:
Urinary Tract Infections

INCIDENCE AND SIGNIFICANCE

Urinary tract infections (UTIs), the most common nosocomial infections, account for a third to a half of all nosocomial bacterial infections. Nearly 15% of hospitalized patients undergo urinary tract catheterization, and more than 90% of nosocomial UTIs are associated with urinary tract catheterization and/or instrumentation. Asymptomatic bacteriuria associated with indwelling catheters, which resolves spontaneously upon removal of the catheter, poses a real problem in defining UTIs. Many would not consider these cases as true UTIs, but they are counted as such by the CDC criteria.[116] If such cases were excluded from the nosocomial UTI rate in our institution, for example, the rate would be reduced by about a third. Bacteremias do occur in such cases, however, and we are inclined to consider them infections until there is better evidence for their insignificance.

Fortunately, most nosocomial UTIs are relatively clinically insignificant and contribute little to morbidity or lengthened hospital stay.[151] Nevertheless, a small but significant percentage of nosocomial UTIs are a major source of septicemia. In our institution, 34% of nosocomial septicemias in which a source could be found were traced to the urinary tract (see Table 7-1). In 1975, the corresponding figure was 27% for 80 hospitals involved in the CDC National Nosocomial Infection Study (NNIS).[115] Such UTIs are associated with lengthened hospital stay, significant morbidity, and occasional mortality. The relation of nosocomial UTIs to the development of pyelonephritis is not well defined.

ETIOLOGIC AGENTS

Escherichia coli is the primary nosocomial pathogen of the urinary tract in all surveillance studies reviewed. Other etiologic microbes commonly encountered include: *Klebsiella pneumoniae*, *Enterobacter* species, *Proteus* species, *Pseudomonas aeruginosa*, *Streptococcus faecalis*, *Staphylococcus epidermidis*, and *Candida albicans*. The relative frequency of various etiologic agents in our institution is reviewed in Table 3-1.

Nosocomial UTIs caused by viruses are generally not well studied and their overall incidence is unknown. Cytomegalovirus involvement in the

19

urinary tract has been well documented, primarily in immunosuppressed patients—especially those who are renal allograft recipients.[596]

TABLE 3-1.—Frequency of Common Pathogens in Nosocomial
Urinary Tract Infections (St. Vincent
Hospital and Medical Center, 1975-1977)

ORGANISM	NUMBER	FREQUENCY (% OF ISOLATES)
Escherichia coli	403	39.0
Streptococcus faecalis (two varieties)	94	9.0
Proteus mirabilis	82	7.9
Pseudomonas aeruginosa	80	7.7
Staphylococcus epidermidis	77	7.4
Klebsiella pneumoniae	64	6.1
Candida albicans	44	4.2
Enterobacter cloacae	23	2.2
Staphylococcus aureus	21	2.0
Streptococcus agalactiae	16	1.5
Torulopsis glabrata	15	1.4
Hemophilus vaginalis	12	1.2
26 other species	108	10.4
Totals	1,039	100.0%

FACTORS AND MECHANISMS OF INFECTION

URINARY CATHETERS

The distal urethra normally is colonized by the skin flora in men and by vulval flora in women. The proximal urethra and urinary bladder are normally sterile. The introduction of a urinary catheter into the bladder provides at least three potential means of microbial entry into this organ.[320]

1. If the catheter is handled improperly prior to catheterization with resultant contamination of the catheter, the catheter itself may be the source of infecting microbes when it is inserted into the bladder.
2. On insertion of the catheter through the urethra, the microbial flora of the anterior urethra are easily picked up by the catheter and thus carried directly into the bladder.
3. In the case of indwelling catheters, the physical presence of the catheter in the urethra provides an abnormal channel between the catheter and

the urethral mucosa for easy passage of microbes from the distal urethra to the bladder. The bladder mucosa and urine are normally maintained sterile by periodic emptying of the bladder via micturition and by the elaboration of antimicrobial secretions by the bladder mucosa. The presence of an indwelling catheter inhibits both of these protective functions. The prevalence of urinary tract colonization and infection increases with the duration of indwelling catheterization.

INSTRUMENTATION AND SURGERY

The most common urinary tract surgical procedure is cystoscopy. Because of the relatively brief stay of the cystoscope in the urethra and the other aseptic techniques used with the procedure, the incidence of UTIs with cystoscopy is much less than that associated with indwelling catheters. Mechanisms of initiating UTIs with instrumentation include the following:

1. Introduction of distal urethral microbes into the bladder during passage of the cystoscope through the urethra into the bladder.
2. Trauma to the urethra from mechanical dilatation during passage of the cystoscope, which renders the mucosa more susceptible to infection and bacteremia. The latter is rarely a problem in the immunologically competent patient since the microbes are rapidly cleared from the bloodstream. In immunocompromised patients, however, this could be a significant threat.
3. Inadequately disinfected or sterilized instruments provide a source and means of exogenous infection of the urinary tract and, in fact, have been the source of nosocomial UTI outbreaks.[415]

SOURCE OF URINARY TRACT PATHOGENS

The source of urinary tract pathogens is usually endogenous, especially in women. The anterior urethra often is contaminated or colonized by microbes from the intestinal tract. These may be introduced into the bladder by the insertion of a catheter or instrument. Exogenous sources, however, also are important and cause most UTI outbreaks. In addition to inadequately disinfected instruments used in urologic surgery mentioned above, exogenous sources include contaminated hands used in inserting catheters or providing catheter care[178, 383, 534] and contaminated vessels used to collect urine from catheters.[640]

PROPHYLACTIC AND CONTROL MEASURES

In attempts to reduce the number of UTIs, most attention has been directed to urinary catheters. Many procedures and devices have been proposed, some of which are effective and some controversial. These have not eliminated the risk, but the risk can be reduced. The basic principles that have been found to be effective in reducing the risk of nosocomial UTIs are the following:

1. Effective hand-washing by personnel between patients.
2. Avoidance of all unnecessary catheterization; this is the most effective measure.
3. Removal of indwelling catheters as soon as possible.
4. Use of sterile technique in the insertion of the catheter. This should include careful cleaning and disinfecting of the periurethral area prior to inserting the catheter. Sterile gloves should be used by the person inserting the catheter.
5. Use of a closed drainage system, which should remain intact and closed throughout the duration of the catheterization. Urine specimens required for tests, including cultures, should be obtained by aspiration from the catheter with a sterile needle and syringe.
6. Good catheter hygiene, including routine perineal, periurethral, and catheter cleansing—both mechanical and with a disinfectant. Sterile gloves should be worn by the person performing this procedure. The establishment of a routine (minimum of twice daily) catheter care procedure in our hospital reduced the number of catheter-associated urinary tract infections by a third.
7. Routine intermittent or continuous irrigation of urinary catheters with various agents has been recommended by many but has not been accepted universally as significantly effective. The triple-lumen catheter should be used for irrigation to maintain the closed drainage system.
8. Use of topical antimicrobics prophylactically is recommended by some but also remains controversial.

The value of the latter two procedures is undoubtedly reduced if the more accepted measures are implemented routinely and effectively. The problem of emerging pathogens that are resistant to many antimicrobics may outweigh any beneficial effects of either form of antimicrobic prophylaxis. Isolation rarely, if ever, plays a role in the control of nosocomial UTIs.

Despite the use of the above precautions, catheter-associated UTIs continue to occur, although at a lower rate than if such precautions are not taken. Many are probably unavoidable given our current understanding of the problem. When an increase in the UTI rate occurs, one must search for common features that might lead to finding a cause, eg, a common organism, common service, or common ward. Such increases are usually due to some breakdown in the prophylactic measures outlined above. Urinary tract infection outbreaks have been traced to faulty insertion techniques and to contaminated disinfectants (especially aqueous benzalkonium chloride), even when supplied in commercially prepared kits.[264] The cause of many UTI outbreaks is never determined specifically, but discussing the problem with the personnel involved often will end the outbreak immediately, presumably due to their increased care and diligence.

Chapter 4:
Respiratory Tract Infections

INCIDENCE AND SIGNIFICANCE

Respiratory tract infections (RTIs) are among the more common nosocomial bacterial infections and may account for as many as 20% of such infections. Lower respiratory tract infections accounted for 15% of the nosocomial infections in 80 NNIS hospitals in 1975.[115]

Nosocomial lower respiratory tract infections are a major cause of deaths that result from nosocomial infections. There is considerable difficulty in assessing the significance of this, however. Many patients with terminal illnesses, especially those with malignancies, develop nosocomial pneumonias that are not aggressively treated, and the patient is allowed to die. For our purposes, it would be more important to know how often nosocomial pneumonias are lethal despite aggressive therapy—a figure that, to my knowledge, is not currently available.

ETIOLOGIC AGENTS

In contrast to community-acquired RTIs, in which *Streptococcus pneumoniae* is the predominant bacterial etiologic agent, nosocomial RTIs are caused more commonly by gram-negative bacilli such as *Klebsiella pneumoniae, Pseudomonas aeruginosa, Serratia marcescens*, and *Escherichia coli.* Table 4–1 gives the relative frequencies of bacterial pathogens in nosocomial RTIs in our institution. Significant differences in the causes of pneumonia have been found in nursing homes as compared with the community at large.[218]

Nosocomial bacterial *infections* of the pharynx and larynx are relatively uncommon. Fungal infection, especially candidal lesions (thrush), are seen with increased frequency in debilitated patients who have malignancies and are receiving immunosuppressant therapy and antibiotics. This accounts for the relatively high incidence of *C albicans* respiratory infections in our hospital (see Table 4–1), which has an active oncology service.

Viral nosocomial RTIs are not uncommon. Undoubtedly, if these were recognized and diagnosed more readily, the incidence of viral nosocomial RTIs would be increased significantly. Hospitals are not spared from community epidemics of viral RTIs such as influenza, and by definition such infections that develop in hospitalized patients are considered nosocomial.

TABLE 4-1.—Frequency of Bacterial and Yeast Pathogens
from Nosocomial Upper and Lower Respiratory
Tract Infections (St. Vincent Hospital
and Medical Center, 1975-1977)

ORGANISM	NUMBER	FREQUENCY (%)
Candida albicans	93	15.1
Escherichia coli	79	12.8
Staphylococcus aureus	72	11.7
Klebsiella pneumoniae	71	11.5
Pseudomonas aeruginosa	41	6.7
Streptococcus pneumoniae	39	6.3
Hemophilus influenzae	38	6.2
Proteus mirabilis	27	4.4
Hemophilus parainfluenzae	20	3.3
Enterobacter cloacae	18	2.9
Enterobacter aerogenes	17	2.8
Acinetobacter calcoaceticus	15	2.4
Serratia marcescens	12	1.9
Torulopsis glabrata	7	1.1
25 other species	67	10.9
Totals	616	100.0%

But outbreaks of viral RTIs in patients confined to hospital wards also occur.[113, 260] In addition, certain nosocomial viral RTIs, eg, cytomegalovirus infections, are particularly likely to occur in debilitated immunosuppressed patients who have malignancies.[404, 437]

Nosocomial parasitic infections, primarily *Pneumocystis carinii* pneumonitis, are seen with increasing frequency—particularly in immunosuppressed patients who have malignancies [472, 565, 634] or organ transplants.[506] Systemic *Strongyloides stercoralis* hyperinfection also occurs primarily in immunosuppressed patients and may involve the lungs.[432, 509]

FACTORS AND MECHANISMS OF RESPIRATORY TRACT INFECTIONS

The source of nosocomial pathogens of the respiratory tract may be either endogenous or exogenous. For endogenous infection, the ultimate source of the pathogen may be the community or the hospital, but in view of the frequency and rapidity with which the upper respiratory tract of hospitalized patients becomes colonized by gram-negative bacilli,[299] it appears that many of the pathogens are of hospital origin. A recent report showed that respiratory tract colonization by gram-negative bacilli in intubated patients and in those who have had a tracheostomy can be traced to gastric overgrowth ($>10^5$/ml) of these microbes—associated with ileus.[25] Exogenous sources are most often associated with nosocomial *epidemics* and have been traced to contaminated aerosols,[249] humidifiers,[249] suction catheters, resuscitation equipment,[69] anesthetic equipment,[444] inhalation therapy nebulizers,[510] tubing,[178] and solutions.[531]

In addition to general systemic factors that increase overall susceptibility to infection, factors that predispose specifically to RTIs include: (1) tracheostomies, (2) respiratory therapy, (3) inhalation anesthesia, (4) endotracheal intubation, and (5) bronchoscopy.

TRACHEOSTOMY

Tracheostomy is a lifesaving, yet relatively simple surgical procedure that is used with increasing frequency in hospitals today, particularly in intensive care units (ICUs). One of the significant risks of this procedure, especially for longer-term tracheostomy patients, is the increased likelihood of respiratory tract infections.

Normally, the respiratory tract below the larynx is sterile or almost so, in contrast with the dense microbial flora in the respiratory tract above the larynx. This sterility is due, at least in part, to the mucus production in the lower respiratory tree, which entraps any microbes that pass through the larynx, and to the ciliary action of the lower respiratory tract mucosa, which keeps the surface blanket of mucus (with entrapped microbes) moving upward toward the mouth. Tracheostomies radically alter this balance of physiologic activity designed to maintain a sterile lower respiratory tract in at least three ways:

1. The trachea is brought into direct continuity with the skin—thus providing an abnormal portal of entry for microbes from the skin and environment into the trachea and totally bypassing the upper respiratory tract. The trachea thus becomes colonized by microbes quite readily, and usually within 24 hours it has developed a microbial flora consisting of cutaneous and upper respiratory tract microbes. If such colonization can be limited to normal cutaneous and pharyngeal flora, infectious complications are relatively uncommon.

2. The presence of the tracheostomy tube injures the tracheal mucosa to varying degrees depending largely on the fit of the tube to the patient's

trachea. The irritation resulting from the tube's presence causes increased mucus production, while the ciliary action of the mucosal cells often is inhibited—resulting in excessive accumulation of tracheal secretions. If points of excessive pressure or friction between the tracheostomy tube and tracheal mucosa develop, ulceration with severe local infection and even perforation may occur.

3. Tracheal toilet is a necessary procedure with a tracheostomy because of the excessive secretions that almost invariably result and the usual absence of the normal mechanisms for removing them. Tracheal toilet refers to tracheal suctioning at intervals sufficient to maintain a patent airway free of excessive secretions. Although tracheal suctioning is essential to tracheostomy care, it is also a significant potential source of infectious complications. Since the suction catheter is introduced into the lower respiratory tree during the suctioning procedure, a contaminated catheter exposes the mucosa to unwanted microbes. There are numerous possibilities for contaminating the catheter with microbes such as *P aeruginosa*, especially in ICUs. Microbes from many environmental sources within the ICU may be carried transiently on the hands of personnel, and their subsequent handling of the tracheal catheter may result in its contamination. Outbreaks of respiratory tract infection in tracheostomy patients are often traced to inadequately cleaned hands of personnel.[153, 375]

RESPIRATORY ASSIST DEVICES

One of the major technical advances in modern medicine has been the development of highly sophisticated respiratory therapy machines, practices, and personnel, which have been effective in the treatment of patients with various respiratory diseases as well as in the prevention of postoperative respiratory complications. During the first few years after the development of these practices, outbreaks of nosocomial RTIs associated with their use were unacceptably common.[86, 88, 178, 289, 510, 652] Most of these outbreaks could be traced to one or more of three problems.

1. Contaminated airways.—The ventilatory apparatus, particularly the tubings and other parts constituting the airway circuit, become contaminated easily and outbreak strains often are cultured from these surfaces.

2. Contaminated humidifiers.—Humidifiers have been used commonly in the airway circuit, particularly for tanked gas such as oxygen (which has no moisture), to prevent excessive drying of the respiratory tract mucosa. Humidifiers frequently were found to be contaminated, often with outbreak strains. The passage of gas through the water in

humidifier canisters not only humidified the gas but also caused the incorporation of microbially contaminated droplet nuclei, which caused subsequent contamination of the airway circuit and the respiratory tract.

3. Contaminated nebulizers.—Nebulizers are devices that atomize solutions into the airway through which droplets of solutions are carried deep into the respiratory tree. They are used primarily as a means of delivering drugs such as mucolytic agents to the respiratory tract. When these are contaminated, they provide a means of delivery of large inocula of microbes via aerosols directly to the alveoli of the lungs. Of the three problems described, contaminated nebulizers pose the greatest single risk of infection.

ANESTHESIA

Inhalation anesthesia shares a number of the infection risks associated with respiratory assist therapy. Outbreaks associated with anesthesia, however, are generally less common.[442] This is undoubtedly due in part to the limited exposure (usually one time only). Nevertheless, the same precautionary measures described for respiratory therapists regarding their equipment should apply to anesthesiologists and anesthetists.

ENDOTRACHEAL TUBES

Endotracheal tubes are useful substitutes for tracheostomies for short periods of time. They are used commonly by anesthesiologists for inhalation anesthesia to ensure that there is an adequate airway. The risk of RTIs associated with endotracheal tubes is considerably less than that with tracheostomies for two reasons: (1) the shorter duration of emplacement (rarely more than one to two days), and (2) the absence of the surgical communications between the trachea and skin. In other respects the two procedures are similar.

BRONCHOSCOPY

Bronchoscopes are tubular instruments used to visualize directly the bronchial tree. Mechanisms of introducing nosocomial RTIs by bronchoscopy include the following:
1. Direct inoculation of the respiratory tract with exogenous microbes by a contaminated instrument. This is most often due to inadequate disinfection of the instrument between uses.
2. Direct inoculation of the lower respiratory tract with endogenous organisms acquired by the bronchoscope during passage through the

upper respiratory tract. The increased colonization of the pharynx by gram-negative bacilli in hospitalized patients, for example, provides a source of potential pathogens to be carried into the bronchial tree by bronchoscopy.[299, 300]

3. Trauma to the respiratory tract mucosa resulting from manipulation of the instrument in the trachea and bronchi. This renders the respiratory tree more susceptible to infection.

PROPHYLACTIC AND CONTROL MEASURES

PROPHYLAXIS

In general, these measures are effective in preventing nosocomial RTIs:

1. Hand-washing by personnel between patient contacts.
2. Effective disinfection or sterilization of components of anesthetic and respiratory therapy equipment that come in contact with respiratory tract mucosa or with gases going to the patient. The use of sterile disposable components is most effective but expensive.
3. The use of sanitary cough techniques by infected patients.

There is little evidence to suggest that isolation of patients with pneumonia is effective in reducing the incidence of nosocomial RTIs when the above procedures are utilized. There are specific instances, however, when isolation of patients with RTIs should be considered, such as a patient who has an open tracheostomy infected with *P aeruginosa* and who is unable to utilize sanitary cough techniques, or a patient with active (open) tuberculosis. There is also little or no evidence to suggest that prophylactic antibiotics are effective for the prevention of nosocomial RTIs.

CONTROL MEASURES

Tracheostomy.—With regard to tracheostomy, the most effective means of prophylaxis against infection is to avoid all unnecessary tracheostomies. Tracheostomies for convenience only are to be condemned. Endotracheal or nasotracheal tubes may suffice as short-term measures, and they present considerably fewer infection risks. Cardiac surgeons who in the past almost routinely performed tracheostomies on patients undergoing open heart surgery have found that most patients can be managed quite adequately without tracheostomies postoperatively. This has resulted in a significant reduction in the number of nosocomial RTIs in this group of patients.

In an attempt to minimize the risk to patients who have tracheostomies, there are two general guidelines: (1) wear disposable sterile gloves when performing tracheal toilet procedures, and (2) use a sterile catheter for suctioning. The latter is accomplished most efficiently by using a new sterile disposable catheter with each suctioning effort. If the catheter must be re-used, thorough cleansing and rinsing in sterile solutions between uses should be standard practice.

Respiratory Assist Devices.—The following are effective control measures:

1. Decontamination of airways.—An effective means of accomplishing this is to use sterile disposable tubing where possible. Ethylene oxide sterilization of all components that are in contact with the air circuit ideally should be done every 24 hours when the components are used for the same patient, or at least between each patient.

2. Humidifiers.—Prophylactic measures include avoidance of un-necessary use of humidifiers and frequent changes of humidifier canisters and water with sterile replacements.

3. Nebulizers.—Prophylactic measures are essentially the same as those for humidifiers. Multientry "sterile" fluids and medication vials should be avoided if possible; if not, they should be replaced with new items at least every eight hours.

When the precautions described above are observed, the risk of RTIs associated with ventilation assist is reduced significantly. The widespread current utilization of these measures has decreased the frequency of RTI outbreaks previously associated with inhalation therapy.

Anesthesia.—The control measures are essentially the same as those for respiratory assist equipment.

Endotracheal Tubes.—Sterile disposable tubes are most desirable from the standpoint of controlling infection, but other practical considerations may dictate the use of reusable tubes. If the latter are used, they should be decontaminated effectively or, preferably, sterilized.

Bronchoscopy.—Bronchoscopes should be sterilized between uses. Because many models will not withstand repeated autoclaving, cold sterilization with agents such as glutaraldehyde should be used.

Chapter 5:
Skin and Wound Infections

The broad group of infections occurring in the skin and wounds includes not only postoperative wound infections but also infections involving burns, decubitus ulcers, and other disease conditions. As many as 25% of the nosocomial infections in general community hospitals may fall into this category.

POSTOPERATIVE WOUND INFECTIONS

INCIDENCE AND SIGNIFICANCE

Postoperative wound infections accounted for 24% of the nosocomial infections in the 80 NNIS hospitals in 1975.[115] These infections should be of primary concern to hospitals because (1) they have significant morbidity and mortality, resulting in significantly prolonged hospitalization, and (2) they are theoretically preventable, at least in clean surgical cases. In assessing postoperative wound infections, it is important to separate cases with an inherent high risk of infection from those without such risk. The following classification by the National Research Council (Altemeier et al, 1968) is useful:

1. Clean surgical cases—crossing no contaminated planes.
2. Clean contaminated cases—in which contaminated areas are entered (eg, bowel) but without gross spillage.
3. Contaminated cases—eg, gross spillage of bowel contents into the peritoneal cavity or recent trauma with external contamination.
4. Infected cases—in which the surgical procedure enters an already infected field, an old traumatic wound, or a field in which a perforated viscus is found.

FACTORS AND MECHANISMS OF INFECTION

The surgical incision is an iatrogenic violation of the skin's integrity. It provides easy access to sterile tissues by surrounding microbes. Until the closed incision heals and is re-epithelialized, it is a weakness in the mechanical barrier—an abnormal portal of entry for microorganisms and a focal area of increased susceptibility to infection.

The source of pathogens in wound infections may be either endogenous or exogenous. During the 1950s and 1960s, when *S aureus* was the primary nosocomial pathogen, many studies implicated the patient's own flora as the source of most *S aureus* wound infections,[660] but others demonstrated the source of some to be exogenous.[42] In category 2, 3, and 4 surgical infections, the source is usually endogenous and the infecting organisms generally are derived from the contaminated or infected area entered. These infections are the most difficult to prevent, but there is some accumulating evidence that prophylactic antibiotics may be beneficial.[121, 126, 307, 351, 481] Exogenous wound infections still occur occasionally, but unless a cluster of infections results, the source usually is not discovered. Epidemics of wound infection continue to be reported and often are traced to a carrier.[27, 253, 424, 535, 584] Anaerobic surgical infections today are almost invariably endogenous.

In addition to the inherent risks mentioned above and systemic alterations in the resistance to infection, factors that have been shown to correlate with an increased prevalence of wound infections include poor surgical technique, increased duration of surgery, high counts of bacteria in the air, penetrated gloves, contaminated instruments, and inadequate disinfection of skin. The corrective measures for such deficiencies are usually obvious and within the capability of any hospital in which surgery is performed. The major difficulty usually is recognizing the deficiency.

ETIOLOGIC AGENTS

Although *S aureus* is still a major wound pathogen, it no longer holds the overwhelming dominance it did 10 to 20 years ago. Gram-negative bacilli such as the Enterobacteriaceae and *P aeruginosa* now equal or surpass *S aureus* in frequency as wound pathogens in most institutions. Although many hypotheses have been proposed to explain this shift, none has been proved and the phenomenon remains poorly understood. Another shift either back to *S aureus* or to some other microbe could occur in the near future. In our institution, for example, the highest frequency of wound infections by gram-negative bacilli occurred in 1975. Whether this is a true peak or a spurious one, only time will tell. The current frequency of postoperative wound pathogens is given in Table 5-1. With improved technology, anaerobes are being recovered with increased frequency from surgical wounds. Although the bandwagon following the new technology may have overemphasized their importance, anaerobes (even in mixed cultures as they usually are) are often significant pathogens. Anaerobes constitute the overwhelming majority of organisms of the normal body flora, and the surprise is the relative infrequency with which they cause infections.

TABLE 5-1.—Frequency of Isolates from Postoperative
Wound Infections (St. Vincent
Hospital and Medical Center, 1975-1977)

ORGANISM	FREQUENCY*	% OF ISOLATES	% OF INFECTIONS
Staphylococcus aureus	129	20.6	32.5
Escherichia coli	116	18.6	29.2
Staphylococcus epidermidis	67	10.7	16.9
Bacterioides fragilis	45	7.2	11.3
Pseudomonas aeruginosa	38	6.1	9.6
Proteus mirabilis	30	4.8	7.6
Streptococcus faecalis (liquefaciens)	25	4.0	6.3
Klebsiella pneumoniae	23	3.7	5.8
Streptococcus faecalis	12	1.9	3.0
Enterobacter cloacae	11	1.8	2.8
Bacillus species	11	1.8	2.8
Non-group A, B, or D Strep. (β)	11	1.8	2.8
Streptococcus agalactiae	10	1.6	2.5
Clostridium perfringens	9	1.4	2.3
Candida albicans	8	1.3	2.0
Corynebacterium species	8	1.3	2.0
Bacteroides melaninogenicus	5	0.8	1.3
Hemophilus vaginalis	5	0.8	1.3
Peptostreptococcus species	5	0.8	1.3
Proteus morgani (Morganella morgani)	5	0.8	1.3
Non-group A, B, or D Strep. (γ)	5	0.8	1.3
Streptococcus pyogenes	5	0.8	1.3
Peptococcus species	4	0.6	1.0
Serratia marcescens	4	0.6	1.0
23 other species	34	5.4	8.6
Totals	625	100.0%	157.8%*

*There were 625 isolates from 397 wound infections—an average of 1.6 isolates per infection. (Isolates present in small numbers were not included.)

PROPHYLACTIC AND CONTROL MEASURES

Prophylactic measures against surgical wound infections focus on preventing microbial access to the incision. Effective procedures in this regard include: (1) thorough cleansing of the skin in and around the operative field before surgery—both mechanical cleansing and the use of effective antiseptic agents are important; (2) similar cleansing of the operating team's hands; (3) use of appropriate surgical drapes; (4) wearing of sterile gloves and gowns by operating personnel; (5) use of thoroughly cleaned and sterile instruments; and (6) postoperative protection of the wound from contamination until the integrity of the skin is reestablished—this usually requires a sterile covering.

Despite the most meticulous care, postoperative wound infections still occur. When such infections occur sporadically with no relation to other infections, the cause or source often remains undetermined. The question: Was it a result of some breakdown in standard procedures, or was it unavoidable by current understanding? usually remains unanswered. On the other hand, when several postoperative wound infections occur and some relationship can be established (eg, common etiologic agent or common physician), then the chances of detecting the source of the problem are enhanced. When such clusters of infections are due to a common microbe, the source can be a carrier who sheds the organism into the environment, as may occur with *S aureus*[424] or *Streptococcus pyogenes*, [253, 393, 535, 584] or the source may be an environmental pathogen such as *Pseudomonas cepacia* that contaminates a disinfectant used for presurgical skin preparation.[41] When no common etiologic agent is found and the evidence points to a particular surgeon, it may be discovered that this surgeon does not observe all the standard procedures such as proper scrub technique or the changing of gloves when they become punctured. When such situations are revealed, the remedial steps needed are usually quite obvious—although it is not always simple to execute them.

Since patients with skin or wound infections often discharge large numbers of infectious organisms into their immediate environment, some form of isolation is recommended to reduce the risk of transmission to other patients or personnel. In the great majority of instances, skin and wound isolation (procedures designed to prevent transmission by direct person-to-person contact) is adequate. Some believe that patients with heavily draining wound infections resulting in frequent dressing saturation, particularly when caused by *S aureus* or *S pyogenes*, should be placed in strict isolation. To my knowledge, however, there is no good evidence that strict isolation is more effective than well-practiced skin and wound isolation in such instances. See the section on isolation in Chapter 8 for more details regarding isolation policies and procedures.

BURNS

Burns invariably become colonized by microbes, and serious and extensive burns almost invariably become infected if prophylactic measures are not taken. Before antibiotics were available, colonizations and infections were predominantly by gram-positive cocci such as *S aureus* and *S pyogenes*, but later colonization and infection were more likely to be due to gram-negative bacilli, particularly *P aeruginosa*.[430] The latter organism has been found to colonize as many as two-thirds of the patients in a burn unit, with the incidence being highest in the patients with more severe burns.[363] The source is usually exogenous. Infected burns are serious infections; they are often prone to dissemination, and in patients who survive the immediate postburn complications, infections are the most common cause of death. Because of this, prophylactic systemic and topical antimicrobics have been used extensively in attempts to reduce the infection rates. The use of the topical agent mafenide (Sulfamylon) has been particularly effective in decreasing infectious complications of burns. One side effect of this, however, has been the increased colonization and infection by fungal agents such as *Candida* and *Aspergillus* species and the Phycomycetes.[200, 429, 430] These also can produce extremely serious infections, but so far the problem is not as great as that of *Pseudomonas* species colonization without prophylaxis.

In the 80 NNIS hospitals reporting nosocomial infections, burn infections accounted for less than 1% of the total infections in 1975.[115] But this varied considerably from hospital to hospital, especially among those with and without burn units, since most seriously burned patients are admitted to hospitals that have burn units. Viral infections of burns also have been reported, especially those due to herpes simplex.[199] Since these infections usually are undiagnosed, it is possible that their frequency is much greater than generally is appreciated. There is some suggestion that herpetic infections of burns may predispose to secondary *P aeruginosa* infection.[199]

Chapter 6:
Other Nosocomial Infections

Although UTIs, RTIs, and skin and wound infections currently account for more than 90% of nosocomial infections, there are other types of nosocomial infections that, despite their relative infrequency, are important because of their severity and/or tendency to occur in epidemics. These will be discussed in detail in this chapter.

GASTROINTESTINAL INFECTIONS

Nosocomial gastrointestinal infections are, fortunately, relatively infrequent compared with the aforementioned infections. There are several types of gastrointestinal infections that are of particular concern to the hospital epidemiologist, eg, epidemic infantile gastroenteritis, salmonellosis, and pseudomembranous colitis.

EPIDEMIC INFANTILE GASTROENTERITIS

Epidemic infantile gastroenteritis is an epidemic diarrheal syndrome that occurs primarily in, but is not limited to, newborn nurseries. The severity varies considerably in different outbreaks, from mild with minimal morbidity to severe with extreme dehydration and mortalities as high as 80%.[248] By far the most common etiologic agent is *Escherichia coli*. Recent studies point to plasmid-mediated enterotoxigenic strains that may or may not belong to the classic, so-called enteropathogenic *E coli* serotypes.[216, 528] Infantile diarrheal outbreaks have occurred, however, in which recognized labile toxins, stable toxins, and invasiveness could not be demonstrated.[357] Host factors, however, must also play a role, which is still poorly understood. For example, why, when all infants in an affected nursery have positive stool cultures, do only some develop the diarrheal syndrome? The striking feature of this disease is its extreme contagiousness despite the most stringent precautions and control measures. Although some outbreaks have been thwarted by such measures as simultaneous treatment of all infants (infected and noninfected) in the nursery with antibiotics such as neomycin, many are not ended until the nursery is closed to new admissions and is thoroughly disinfected.

SALMONELLOSIS

This gastrointestinal infection is caused by any of more than 1,000 serotypes of *Salmonella enteritidis* that may become systemic by bloodstream invasion—so-called enteric fever—and in turn may result in death. Nosocomial salmonellosis may be sporadic, usually resulting from contact with an infected patient. More important and striking are nosocomial salmonellosis outbreaks, which usually involve both patients and hospital personnel. Two modes of transmission are recognized. The first is foodborne outbreaks, which are the most dramatic and tend to be large outbreaks. Rapid recognition of the outbreak followed by intense epidemiologic investigation with identification of the culprit food item is essential for the timely containment of such outbreaks. Most foodborne nosocomial salmonellosis outbreaks have been traced to contaminated eggs or egg products.[541] The second mode is person-to-person transmission, which tends to result in smaller, more insidious outbreaks that are often much more difficult to solve epidemiologically. The transmission is via the fecal-oral contamination route, and the source is usually one or more asymptomatic carriers of the incriminated strain.[365, 541] Some outbreaks may begin as foodborne outbreaks; after removal of the responsible food source, the outbreak may drag on due to subsequent person-to-person spread.[586] Unusual means of transmission are encountered occasionally, eg, endoscopy with inadequate decontamination of the instrument following use on an infected index patient.[122]

PSEUDOMEMBRANOUS COLITIS

Also referred to as antibiotic-associated colitis, pseudomembranous colitis has received considerable attention recently because of its association with clindamycin usage. Recent studies on the feces of patients with pseudomembranous colitis have demonstrated the presence of a toxin that is cytotoxic to human amnion cells and produces enterocolitis in hamsters. This toxin is neutralized by *Clostridium sordellii* and *C difficile* antitoxins.[40, 224, 346, 507] *C difficile*, but not *C sordellii*, frequently has been isolated from the feces of such patients, and it produces a toxin indistinguishable from that in patients' feces.[224, 347] Furthermore, *C difficile* is resistant to clindamycin,[40] and because of the susceptibility of most anaerobes to this drug, the administration of clindamycin may permit or encourage a relative overgrowth of *C difficile* with increased toxin production and colitis. Pseudomembranous colitis, a severe iatrogenic illness, has caused the deaths of some persons and has required colectomies to save others. If further studies support the role of *C difficile* and its toxin in the etiology of this dread complication, vancomycin would appear to be the drug of choice in treatment—based on studies in hamsters.[347]

MISCELLANEOUS INFECTIONS

Miscellaneous gastroenteric infections occur sporadically as well as in outbreaks in the hospital setting. Drug-related diarrheas may be difficult to differentiate from infectious diarrheas of viral etiology since bacterial enteric pathogens are absent in both. Viral cultures may be helpful in making such differential diagnoses but often are not practical. In an outbreak the differential diagnosis is usually easier. Nosocomial outbreaks of viral gastroenteritis are well recognized.[91, 125, 340] In many patients, infectious diarrhea is assumed to be of viral origin in the absence of bacterial enteropathogens and parasites, but only rarely are these assumptions ever proved. Many gram-negative bacilli that are considered normal intestinal residents may occasionally produce significant enteric disease—particularly in neonates and infants. These pathogens include commonly isolated microbes such as *Proteus* species and *P aeruginosa*.[176] *Yersinia enterocolitica* and *Edwardsiella tarda* are probably true enteric pathogens and are not to be considered normal flora.[70, 305, 611]

HEPATITIS

Hepatitis is generally of viral etiology when due to a microbial agent. Often the clinical picture is indistinguishable from that of drug-associated hepatitis, such as that associated with halothane anesthesia. From the standpoint of infection control, it is safest to assume that all cases of hepatitis and jaundice are of viral etiology until proved otherwise; ie, the same precautions should be taken as for known viral hepatitis. Many viruses are capable of causing hepatitis. Hepatitis B virus in the past was a major cause of transfusion-associated hepatitis, but the prevalence of this form of hepatitis has been reduced significantly by the exclusion of donor blood that is positive for the HB_s antigen. However, dialysis-associated hepatitis B still remains a significant nosocomial problem (see the next section). Hepatitis A virus is rarely a cause of transfusion hepatitis and is more likely to be transmitted by the fecal-oral route. Hepatitis C virus, which may be more than one agent, is responsible for most cases of transfusion-related hepatitis encountered today. (A more detailed description of these three agents can be found in Chapter 9.) In addition to these agents, however, several others have been shown to cause nosocomial viral hepatitis. These include cytomegalovirus,[193, 596] Epstein-Barr virus,[131] and herpes simplex virus,[519] all of which are DNA viruses and which produce such infections mainly in immunosuppressed patients. The actual incidence of nosocomial viral hepatitis is difficult to assess because the long incubation period results in such infections becoming manifest after patients are discharged from the hospital. Most hospital epidemiology programs have found surveillance of postdischarge nosocomial infections very difficult and frustrating. Occasionally bacterial etiologies of hepatitis are encountered, eg, granulomatous hepatitis due to bacille Calmette Guérin (BCG) in patients with cancer who receive BCG immunotherapy.[286, 523, 545]

DIALYSIS-ASSOCIATED INFECTIONS

Hemodialysis has been associated with nosocomial infection. In recent years much attention has centered on hepatitis B virus in hemodialysis units, which poses a threat not only to patients but also to attending personnel.[221, 370] Based on a CDC survey of 65 dialysis units, it was calculated that the incidence of infection caused by hepatitis B virus was 4.4 per 100 hemodialysis patients and 3.4 per 100 dialysis unit personnel.[221] Where possible, it would appear prudent to employ personnel for work in dialysis units who are HB_S-antibody-positive, and thus theoretically resistant to hepatitis B virus. Other agents also have been incriminated in outbreaks related to hemodialysis, including Epstein-Barr virus,[131] *Citrobacter* and *Flavobacterium* species,[582] *P aeruginosa*,[621, 632] *Salmonella* species,[582] *S marcescens*,[582] *S aureus*,[331] and even *Bacillus* species.[138] Most of these infections are sepsis or shunt infections.

Peritoneal dialysis also is associated with an increased risk of nosocomial infections—primarily peritonitis. Since many of these patients are on antibiotic therapy, the incidence of candida peritonitis is particularly high in this group of patients.[165, 197, 644] One report suggests that there is increased risk of infection by hepatitis B virus in patients in peritoneal dialysis units also.[576]

INFECTIONS ASSOCIATED WITH INTRAVASCULAR DEVICES

The insertion of intravenous (IV) lines (catheters or needles) is second in frequency only to phlebotomies among invasive procedures performed on hospitalized patients. In the average acute care hospital, as many as 50% of patients will have an IV line in place sometime during their hospitalization. Because they are so commonplace, their potential as a source of nosocomial infection often is regarded too lightly.

Not only do IV lines provide a break in the normal mechanical barrier or defense of the skin, but they also provide a direct conduit from the environment to the bloodstream. Consequently, microbes of the cutaneous flora and the environment as well as contaminated fluids have easy access to the internal milieu of the body. This may result in one or more of the following: colonization and infection of the IV site, colonization of the intravascular segment of the IV line, bacteremia with or without sepsis and seeding of other tissues, septic phlebitis, and purulent thrombophlebitis. Many of these complications are serious and potentially lethal. It has been estimated that intravenous infusions account for 35,000 cases of septicemia annually in the United States, with a death rate of about 30%.[582] Numerous factors have been identified as being important in affecting the risk of developing intravascular device infections. Some important ones are listed here.

INSERTION SITE

In general, IV sites in the lower extremity are more likely to become infected than those in the upper extremity—presumably due to the differences in cutaneous microbial flora and contamination. Intravenous lines through injured (eg, burned) skin are far more prone to infection than those through healthy skin. Intravenous sites in close proximity to cutaneous eruptions or infections (eg, eczema, furuncles) result in more infections than lines more distant from such sites. Such information means that the site of insertion is important and must be selected carefully.

INSERTION PROCEDURE

There are few factual data to indicate that the actual technique of insertion is a significant determinant of whether subsequent colonizations or infections occur. In our study, no difference in colonization rates occurred between lines that were easy or difficult to insert.[211] Nevertheless, there are rational reasons for accepting certain procedures in the insertion of IV lines, such as: (1) thorough cleansing and disinfection of the skin at and around the proposed site; (2) thorough hand-washing by the operator and, depending on circumstances, wearing of sterile gloves; and (3) use of sterile disposable needles, which should be discarded after the first penetration of the skin; ie, a needle should not be reused if the first attempt at cannulation fails. The choice of antiseptic for skin preparation is important. Agents such as aqueous benzalkonium chloride are not recommended because they are readily contaminated by and support the growth of organisms such as *Pseudomonas cepacia*. Aqueous benzalkonium chloride has been shown to be a source of nosocomial bacteremias when it is used to prepare the skin for intravenous infusion.[208] Iodophors and alcohol are preferable.

CATHETER CARE

Catheter neglect is probably the single most important factor allowing the development of infections associated with IV lines. Appropriate catheter care means frequent (at least twice daily), careful examination of the IV catheter system and insertion site, with immediate removal of the line at the first signs of problems or difficulties, such as pain at the catheter site, leakage of infusion fluid around the needle, subcutaneous infiltration, or phlebitis. Colonization of IV lines occurs significantly more frequently in such "problem" lines than in lines without such difficulties.[211] Hence, the best defense is the removal of the IV line as soon as or before such problems develop.

DURATION OF CATHETERIZATION

The exact role of the duration of catheter emplacement is still in some dispute. There is universal agreement that the longer the catheter is in, the more likely colonization and infection will occur. The controversial point, however, is the nature of this relationship, ie, is it linear or logarithmic? This is of more than academic interest since the recommended procedure of changing lines every 48 hours is based on studies that show a significant increase in colonization and infection of catheters that are in place longer than 48 hours.[382] On the other hand, some studies have shown that the relationship is linear,[211] ie, the risk of colonization of a catheter in place for two days is twice as great as that of a catheter in for one day, and one in place for ten days has ten times more risk of colonization than one in for one day, etc. If such a relationship exists, there is no advantage to frequent changing of catheters since the risk of infection would not be altered. In fact, such frequent changes may be detrimental from the standpoint of patient discomfort; many patients who require prolonged IV infusions are seriously ill and are often difficult to cannulate.

It is our opinion, after carefully reviewing the literature and our own experiences, that the critical factor is catheter care. Institutions in which frequent catheter monitoring is not possible should adopt the recommendation of routinely changing IV lines every two days. In those institutions in which good catheter care policies are practiced (best accomplished by a dedicated IV team), the duration of normal function without problems or complications can be used to determine the frequency of catheter change.

PLASTIC CANNULAE VERSUS NEEDLES

The use of plastic cannulae for IV infusions has increased in recent years because they permit greater patient comfort and longer duration of use and because of the increased ease with which they now can be inserted. Many investigators indicate that the use of plastic cannulae results in more infections than occur with the use of steel needles and recommend minineedles (scalp vein needles) for long-term IV infusion.[382] However, at least two studies have shown that colonization of such minineedles is quite frequent in patients with malignancies.[367, 376] In another study no appreciable difference in colonization rates for plastic and scalp vein needles was observed after six days.[473]

INFUSION PRODUCTS

It is axiomatic that all efforts must be made to ensure the sterility of infusion products. The potential for contamination of such products is great and can be caused by inadequate sterilization of the product or its containers, subsequent contamination in the manufacturing process, contamination when entering containers for the purpose of making mixtures or adding drugs, and other poor techniques. Although most infusion products are prepared commercially today, this has not provided a guarantee against contamination. Well documented nationwide outbreaks of bacteremia and sepsis have occurred due to contaminated commercial infusion products.[102, 190] Fortunately, these have been rare but have provided one of the justifications for widespread hospital infection surveillance programs. Two infusion products, high-calorie nutrients and blood products, require further comment.

Intravenous Hyperalimentation.—High-calorie nutritional solutions can be prepared for intravenous use and may be substituted temporarily for normal alimentary nutrition. The process of preparation of these solutions along with the tailoring of the recipe to the individual patient is becoming a sophisticated technical science. In most institutions, such solutions are prepared by the pharmacy department. Because of the complexity of these solutions, the potential for contamination is great. The seriousness of such contamination is magnified by the highly nutritious nature of the solutions, which enhances the rapid growth of many microbes. Furthermore, gross contamination of such solutions may be difficult to detect since counts of 10^5 bacteria or more per milliliter may be present with no detectable change in the appearance of the solution. Yeast colonization and infection has been a serious problem associated with intravenous hyperalimentation.[24, 453, 622, 644]

Efforts to control the problem center on both the careful preparation of the solutions and meticulous insertion and maintenance of the IV line through which the solution is infused. The solution should be prepared in as clean an area as possible, preferably in a laminar flow hood. The components should be sterile, and aseptic techniques must be maintained throughout.

Blood and Blood Products.—This form of infusion product, which cannot be subjected to the usual sterilization procedures, continues to be a significant source of nosocomial infection. The screening of blood and blood donors for infective microbes and the rejection of such units remain a major challenge for blood banks. Until recently this has been accomplished primarily by taking the histories of prospective donors and rejecting those who have had certain illnesses such as hepatitis, jaundice, or malaria. Undoubtedly, this has lowered the number of transfusion-related infections. The recent practice of routinely screening all units of blood for HB_sAg and rejecting those that are antigen-positive has reduced markedly the incidence of transfusion-induced infection by hepatitis B virus.[15]

Other forms or causes of transfusion-associated hepatitis persist as significant problems. Almost any infectious process in which there is a bloodborne phase can be transmitted by blood or blood product transfusion. In many instances the infected person may be clinically well during this period, and blood donated at this time is accepted. For example, viremias may occur in asymptomatic carriers (eg, hepatitis B virus) or during the prodrome of many viral infections prior to onset of clinical illness. Transfusion-associated infections, however, are not limited to viruses, since documented instances of rickettsial, bacterial, and protozoal transmissions are recorded. Examples are listed in Table 6-1.

PRESSURE TRANSDUCERS

Increasingly, seriously ill patients are being monitored by a variety of devices with direct intravascular communications, eg, continuous blood pressure monitoring devices. Contaminated pressure transducers have been reported on several occasions to be sources of nosocomial outbreaks.[103, 131, 475] Despite the inconvenience it may pose, effective sterilization of such devices between uses is indicated, eg, ethylene oxide sterilization.

INTRA-ARTERIAL CATHETERS

Although not used as frequently as intravenous catheters, indwelling arterial catheters are being used increasingly, particularly in critically ill patients. They are subject to the same risks as IV lines; infections and even outbreaks have been traced to their use.[583]

In conclusion, the use of intravascular infusions, implements, and devices has brought about major advances in diagnostic and therapeutic technology but has also provided microbes with portals of entry directly to the bloodstream, against which appropriate precautions and vigilance must be directed.

TABLE 6-1.—Examples of Nosocomial Infections
Acquired Via Transfusions

MICROBES	REFERENCES
Cytomegalovirus	309, 488
Hepatitis B virus	142, 152, 487
Hepatitis non-A, non-B virus	183, 282, 401, 487
Rickettsia burnetii	108
Rickettsia rickettsii	647
Salmonella choleraesuis	503
Serratia marcescens	67
Plasmodium species	123, 149, 220, 547
Toxoplasma gondii (?)	524

MENINGITIS

Meningitis is a serious, but fortunately relatively uncommon type of nosocomial infection, accounting for less than 0.5% of nosocomial infections in NNIS hospitals.[115] Nosocomial meningitis occurs most often in neonates, and the two most common etiologic agents are *Streptococcus agalactiae* (group B streptococci)[36] and *Escherichia coli*.[391,511] These organisms may be acquired by an infant during passage through the colonized birth canal of the mother or after delivery by contact with carriers, eg, mother or nursing personnel. *Listeria monocytogenes* also characteristically causes neonatal meningitis, but this condition is always acquired from the mother and is relatively uncommon in the United States. Outbreaks of nosocomial meningitis are seldom caused by the aforementioned organisms, but rather are due to microbes such as *Flavobacterium meningosepticum*,[380,479] *Citrobacter diversus*,[251,257,509] and *Proteus mirabilis*,[85,561] which may be found as contaminants in the nursery environment. Such outbreaks may be extremely difficult to unravel.

CEREBROSPINAL FLUID SHUNT INFECTIONS

Shunts from the ventricular system of the brain to the vascular system, such as ventriculoatrial shunts, are being used increasingly to relieve conditions of increased cerebrospinal fluid pressure. Such shunts are in place for very long periods of time and are susceptible to infections by cutaneous flora microbes of relatively low pathogenicity, such as *Staphylococcus epidermidis*.[495]

INFECTIONS ASSOCIATED WITH ENDOSCOPY

Endoscopes are flexible (eg, fiberoptic scopes) or inflexible (usually metal) tubular instruments used for direct visualization of internal hollow structures that are not otherwise accessible without invasion. These include such common instruments as bronchoscopes, gastroscopes, sigmoidoscopes, colonoscopes, and cystoscopes. Cystoscopy and bronchoscopy have been discussed briefly in preceding chapters. Nosocomial infections associated with endoscopy may occur by at least two mechanisms: cross-infection and endogenous infection.

CROSS-INFECTION

There are many well documented instances of infections and infection outbreaks traceable to endoscopy of the respiratory tract, gastrointestinal tract, and genitourinary tract. These are almost always due to inadequate decontamination of instruments between uses or to the use of contaminated disinfectants for decontaminating the instruments. Ideally, these instruments should be sterilized between uses, but many will not withstand the stresses of autoclaving. Consequently, cold sterilization must be used, and agents such as glutaraldehyde have been found to be effective. Agents such as an aqueous solution of benzalkonium chloride or chlorhexidine should not be used because microbes such as strains of *P aeruginosa*, *P cepacia*, and some Enterobacteriaceae may be resistant and actually reproduce in them.

ENDOGENOUS INFECTIONS

The concept of endogenous infections associated with endoscopy is based on few facts and many theoretical considerations. Clearly, the passage of an endoscope through a colonized passage (eg, upper respiratory tract and urethra) prior to entry into a normally sterile region (eg, bronchial tree and urinary bladder) introduces microbes into these susceptible areas. If potential pathogens are included in these flora, the risk of infection is increased. The increased colonization of the pharynx by gram-negative bacilli in hospitalized patients,[299, 300] for example, provides a source of potential pathogens to be carried into the bronchial tree by bronchoscopy. Some endoscopic procedures result in mechanical dilatation of the passages through which the endoscope traverses (eg, cystoscopes and sigmoidoscopes). When such passages are heavily colonized by microbial flora, as is the anal mucosa, or are infected (eg, in urethritis and prostatitis), the resulting trauma to the respective mucosae provides easy access of microbes to the bloodstream. Bacteremias following such procedures are well documented. In immunologically competent patients, this appears to pose no problem, since the bloodstream is cleared of the bacteria within 30 minutes after the procedure. In compromised patients, however, the risk is more substantial. Prophylactic measures against this type of complication are difficult to recommend in the absence of data. On theoretical grounds, the use of prophylactic antimicrobics during endoscopy procedures in high-risk patients may be justifiable.

INFECTIONS ASSOCIATED WITH PHLEBOTOMY

The use of evacuated tubes in phlebotomies for the procurement of blood specimens is now standard practice in most USA hospitals. Although these commercially prepared evacuated tubes are not guaranteed sterile, no potential infection threat had been recognized in association with this practice until recently. A recent report demonstrated that a significant proportion of the evacuated tubes are, in fact, contaminated,[638] and instances have been reported of bacteremia and pseudobacteremia caused by their use.[104, 394] Although the risk of infection from the use of these tubes—particularly if the manufacturer's instructions and recommendations are followed—is quite minimal, the use of recently available sterile evacuated tubes should essentially eliminate this risk. Another variation on this theme is the so-called pseudobacteremia following phlebotomies for blood culture; it is due to contamination of the antiseptic used for cleansing the skin.[316] In such instances, the blood cultures are positive for the same microbes that contaminate the antiseptic, but no true bacteremia exists. However, three of 38 patients in one such episode apparently did develop true bacteremia through exposure in this manner.[316]

INFECTIONS ASSOCIATED WITH PROSTHETIC DEVICES

Here we refer mainly to prosthetic joints and heart valves. Total hip replacements have received considerable acceptance in recent years and are associated with an extremely low infection rate—less than 1%. When such rare infections occur, however, they can be devastating. There is almost universal agreement that prophylactic antimicrobial therapy is justified in this type of surgery. Despite such prophylaxis, however, occasional prosthesis infections occur months or even years after surgery; these are caused by microbes of relatively low pathogenicity, such as *S epidermidis*. There is considerable controversy regarding the source of these infections, but the two most probable hypotheses are the following: (1) Infection occurs at the time of surgery, and the implanted microbe either remains latent until more favorable conditions develop or produces its damaging effects so slowly that they take months to become clinically manifest. (2) Infection occurs as a result of seeding from transient bacteremias, and because of the presence of the foreign body, local tissue reactions are unable to eradicate it. If the former instance is true, such infections would be nosocomial. It is possible that both mechanisms may be involved.

Infective endocarditis involving prosthetic cardiac valves is a well-recognized complication of valve replacement. Infections may become manifest in the immediate postoperative period or many months later. It is probable that the more immediate infections occur at the time of surgery, whereas the mechanism of the late-onset infections involves the two hypotheses mentioned above for orthopedic prostheses. The etiologic agents of prosthetic valve endocarditis are generally quite different from those of the more usual infective endocarditis. They tend to be organisms of relatively low pathogenicity, but are often resistant to the commonly used antimicrobial prophylactic agents, eg, *Candida* species,[642] *Aspergillus* species,[156, 308, 349] *S epidermidis*,[120, 578] corynebacteria,[225, 302] and even atypical mycobacteria.[17, 369] Prosthetic valve endocarditis is often refractory to medical therapy alone and may require replacement surgery as well.

INFECTIONS ASSOCIATED WITH MISCELLANEOUS PROCEDURES

Several additional invasive procedures are common today in hospital practice; some of these have been associated with rare infections but to date have not presented such significant problems as those described above. Examples include cardiac catheterization,[530] bone marrow aspiration, and needle biopsies of the liver, kidney, lung, and other organs. One relatively new procedure enjoying current popularity is intrapartum fetal monitoring utilizing fetal scalp electrodes. Recent studies indicate that the infection rate (scalp abscesses) following this procedure is significant and may be as high as 4.5%.[350, 443, 617] If these reports are substantiated, this practice will become another significant nosocomial infection problem.

There are a host of hospital articles and procedures that have been implicated as rare sources of nosocomial infection, or have been evaluated and concluded to be potential sources of infection. They include thermometers, stethoscopes, electrocardiographic leads, and blood pressure cuffs, among others. With the standard cleaning procedures used in most hospitals, these articles have little threat as sources of infection—although they shouldn't be totally ignored. It is important to remember that many commercially prepared items used on patients may erroneously be assumed to be sterile. When used for the purpose for which they are intended, however, they are rarely associated with problems. This is illustrated by the recently reported outbreaks of *Rhizopus* species wound infections and abscesses associated with the use of commercial adhesive elastic bandages, which subsequently were shown to be contaminated with this organism.[109, 112] Unusual infections should raise the possibilities of unusual sources.

In effect, almost any body site or organ may become involved in a nosocomial infection under appropriate circumstances. Examples not mentioned to this point include puerperal sepsis,[298] neonatal tetanus,[344] encephalitis,[570] endophthalmitis,[165, 197, 644] osteomyelitis,[85, 360] and septic arthritis.[240]

INFECTIONS ASSOCIATED WITH CARRIERS

Patients who are colonized persistently by potentially pathogenic microbes may be sources for nosocomial infections—both sporadic and epidemic. Nosocomial outbreaks occasionally traced to such carriers may be due to many different species; eg, *S aureus*,[27, 424] *S pyogenes*,[253, 298, 393, 535, 584] *Salmonella* species,[541] *P mirabilis*,[85] or hepatitis B virus.[79, 522, 576] Carriage may be nasal, pharyngeal, intestinal, anal, vaginal, cutaneous, or bloodborne. In most instances the risk of dissemination to others virtually can be eliminated by the practice of the standard hygiene policies recommended in hospitals. Rare carriers may be "disseminators" or "shedders," whereby (via viral interaction?)[168, 184] large numbers of microbes are shed into the environment—even airborne. Such carriers are hazardous, and elimination of the carrier state is essential before allowing such persons to work in patient care areas.

HAND TRANSMISSION OF INFECTIONS

Probably the most important means of transmission of infections from person to person are people's hands. The hands normally are colonized by the usual skin flora, which constitutes the resident skin flora of the hands. Because of the conscious and unconscious explorative tendency of the hands, they are in frequent contact with other parts of the body (notoriously the face, nose, and mouth) as well as myriads of objects in the environment, including other people. In the process of these tactile explorations, hands acquire additional microbes from these many points of contact. These constitute a rather transitional type of flora, which are just as readily deposited on subsequent items of contact. In this manner, the hand becomes an efficient means of transferring microbes from person to person, from person to fomites, from fomites to person, and so on. Countless possibilities of cross-infection by hands in the hospital setting easily can be imagined and are very real. Hands have been implicated as the means of transmission in a large number of nosocomial outbreaks.[381] Hands may play a significant role in the person-to-person transfer of upper respiratory viral infections such as the common cold.[256]

The transient flora of the hands are of major importance in cross-infection. These flora are removed effectively by hand-washing, which thus provides an effective means of breaking the chain of microbial transfer by hands. Despite its ease, ready availability, and proved effectiveness, hand-washing is still a commonly neglected practice—even among physicians, nurses, and other health care personnel. Hand-washing between all patient contacts should be automatic for all health care personnel and, if universally practiced, would undoubtedly have a greater impact on lowering the nosocomial infection rate than any other currently known infection control measure.

Chapter 7:
Bacteremia

For purposes of this chapter, the term *bacteremia* also includes fungemia. Between 5% and 10% of nosocomial infections are associated with a bacteremia. In a three-year period (1975-1977), bacteremias occurred in 8% of the nosocomial infections in our institution, and in 1975 they occurred in about 7% of the nosocomial infections reported by 80 NNIS hospitals.[115] Approximately half of these infections occur without any clinical or microbiologic identifiable source and are referred to as *primary bacteremias*. Those in which a primary infection site is identified as the source of the bacteremia are referred to as *secondary bacteremias*. The source distribution of nosocomial bacteremias experienced in our institution from 1975 to 1977 is shown in Table 7-1. Although urinary tract infections are the most common source of secondary bacteremias, the incidence of bacteremias secondary to UTIs is the lowest of the groups listed. Intravenous cannulae infections are associated with the highest incidence of bacteremias.

The term *primary bacteremia* is a cover-up for our inability to track down the source of a bacteremia. We have examined some epidemiologic variables surrounding nosocomial bacteremias in an attempt to find epidemiologic differences between primary and secondary bacteremias. Figure 7-1 shows that the frequencies of both primary and secondary bacteremias by age of patient are essentially identical, with the peak frequency of both occurring in the seventh decade. No appreciable difference in the sex of patients was observed. Ninety-seven percent of the patients with nosocomial bacteremias had IV lines at the time of infection, with no difference between primary and secondary bacteremias, and 94% of these patients had urinary catheters, again with no significant difference between the two bacteremia types. Sixty-four percent of patients with nosocomial bacteremias were receiving antibiotics at the time of infection, but only a third of these had secondary bacteremias. Similarly, only a third of the bacteremias in patients receiving corticosteroid and/or immunosuppressant chemotherapy were secondary. Sixty-nine percent of patients with nosocomial bacteremias were on the surgical services, and of these, only 38% were primary bacteremias; in contrast, of the medical patients who developed nosocomial bacteremias, 64% were primary.

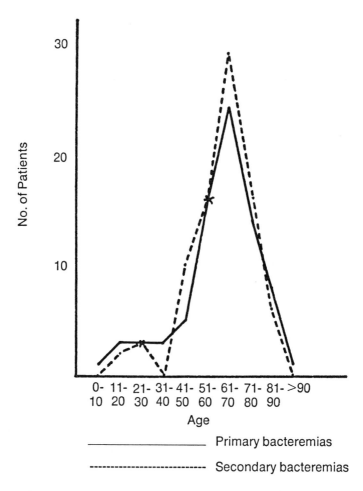

Fig 7-1. Bacteremias associated with age of patient. (St. Vincent Hospital and Medical Center, 1975-1977.)

It is apparent that patients who develop nosocomial bacteremias are seriously ill and consistently require intravenous and urinary catheterization. Patients who develop primary bacteremia differ from those who develop secondary bacteremia in that they are more likely to be receiving antibiotics at the time or immediately prior to the onset of the bacteremia. If patients who are receiving corticosteroids or chemotherapy develop nosocomial bacteremia, it is two times more likely to be primary bacteremia than secondary.

TABLE 7-1.—Sources of Nosocomial Bacteremias
(St. Vincent Hospital and Medical Center, 1975-1977)

SOURCE	NUMBER	% OF BACTEREMIAS	% BY SOURCE*
Unknown (primary)	75	49	—
Known (secondary)	79	51	—
Urinary tract	27	34	2.7
Respiratory tract	17	22	3.3
Postoperative wounds	15	19	3.8
IV cannulae	13	16	28.3
Miscellaneous	7	9	4.6

*Percent of specific infections associated with bacteremias.

Autopsy studies of several patients who died during or shortly after their primary bacteremic episodes often fail to identify a focus of infection as the source. However, a common feature of many cases is the presence of gastrointestinal lesions such as ulcerations secondary to tumor infiltrates, chemotherapy, or fungal infections. These lesions exposed to the heavy normal flora of the gut would appear to provide easy access for microbes into the bloodstream. This mechanism undoubtedly accounts for a significant number of primary bacteremias, particularly in patients with various malignancies who are being treated with steroids and chemotherapy.

In general, the frequency of various pathogens isolated from the blood parallels the frequency with which they are found in three major types of infection—UTIs, RTIs, and wound infections. Hence, in our series from 1975 to 1977 (Table 7-2), S aureus and E coli are isolated with equal frequency and lead the list.

TABLE 7-2.—Frequency of Isolates from Nosocomial Bacteremias
(St. Vincent's Hospital and Medical Center, 1975–1977)

ORGANISM	FREQUENCY			% OF ISOLATES*
	PRIMARY	SECONDARY	TOTAL	
Staphylococcus aureus	13	13	26	16.0
Escherichia coli	6	19	25	15.3
Bacterioides fragilis	6	10	16	9.8
Klebsiella pneumoniae	7	7	14	8.6
Pseudomonas aeruginosa	6	8	14	8.6
Candida albicans	7	5	12	7.4
Staphylococcus epidermidis	5	7	12	7.4
Serratia marcescens	3	2	5	3.1
Streptococcus viridans	3	1	4	2.5
Acinetobacter calcoaceticus	3	—	3	1.8
Streptococcus pneumoniae	1	2	3	1.8
Proteus mirabilis	2	1	3	1.8
Torulopsis glabrata	1	2	3	1.8
Citrobacter freundii	1	1	2	1.2
Streptococcus faecalis	1	1	2	1.2
Streptococcus faecalis (*liquefaciens*)	1	1	2	1.2
17 species with one each	9	8	17	10.4
Totals	75	88	163	99.9%

*Figures are rounded to the nearest 0.1%.

Chapter 8:
Epidemiology Program

In the previous seven chapters, the problems of nosocomial infections, some of the factors influencing them, and the nature of such infections have been reviewed briefly in the light of our current understanding. We draw the following conclusions: (1) From the standpoint of patient morbidity and mortality, as well as economic cost to the community, nosocomial infections present a major problem. (2) From our present understanding of the factors causing, predisposing to, and influencing nosocomial infections, it is apparent that some infections are clearly preventable. (3) It therefore behooves health care facilities to take all reasonable steps possible to keep the number of nosocomial infections to a minimum.

In this section the principles and some practical approaches to hospital epidemiology and infection control will be presented. Specific policies and procedures outlined in this chapter are those currently used at the author's institution. Although the basic concept and principles are applicable to most or all health care institutions, the specific approaches may and should vary among individual facilities. Not only are there major differences in types of institutions (county hospitals, Veterans Administration hospitals, community hospitals, and extended care facilities), but also within any given type, no two facilities are identical in all respects. Consequently, the methodological approach to infection control must be tailored to the individual requirements and peculiarities of each health care facility.

GENERAL ASPECTS OF INFECTION CONTROL PROGRAMS

All nosocomial infection epidemiology programs must have two essential components in order to be effective: (1) a means of assessing infection in the institution (commonly referred to as *surveillance*) and (2) a means of implementing effective control measures. Either alone is almost without value. The most sophisticated surveillance system contributes little if there is no means of taking appropriate remedial action in response to problems. Likewise, the significance of the most stringent procedures designed to control infections is indeterminable when there is no means of surveillance to assess the preexisting state and the effect of the control procedures. A third component of great importance implied in the term *surveillance* is a means of appropriate analysis of surveillance data. This is an essential nexus between the other two components. In my experience it is the most common deficit in unsuccessful epidemiology programs. The best surveillance data together with all the necessary authority to implement control measures remain ineffective unless there is also salient analysis to give appropriate direction to the control measures.

PERSONNEL

For any hospital epidemiology program to be effective it is essential that there be appropriate personnel to operate the program.

NURSE EPIDEMIOLOGIST

The majority of people who occupy this position are nurses and hence are often referred to as infection control nurses or nurse epidemiologists (NE). However, a significant number are not nurses (and it is not necessary that they be), and therefore the term *infection control practitioner* has been proposed. Since all hospital personnel should be "practitioners" of infection control, we believe this is a poor term. Consequently, despite its admitted shortcomings, the term *nurse epidemiologist* will be used hereafter. It is important that the NE be qualified, capable, and willing to carry out the function of this position. In addition to having basic understanding of infections, epidemiology, and infection control (particularly in a hospital setting), it is extremely important that the NE be able to develop good rapport with and gain the trust of physicians, nursing personnel, all other personnel, and the administration. It should be apparent from the duties listed below that much of the information to which NEs have access is confidential, thus making discretion and tact important qualifications of NEs.

The NE is the central thread around which the infection control program is woven. Among the primary duties and responsibilities of the NE in our hospital are the following:
1. To monitor infection.
2. To make regular ward rounds to obtain data on infected patients.
3. To identify the source and method of transmission of each nosocomial infection whenever possible.
4. To distinguish between nosocomial infections and community-acquired infections.
5. To monitor admitting and microbiologic data closely to detect patients that have nosocomial infections from previous admissions.
6. To order or obtain wound cultures (from purulent draining wounds) if not already ordered by a physician. The patient's physician should be notified of this, however.
7. To maintain complete records on all patients with infections.

8. To conduct specific investigations to determine the existence of outbreaks within the hospital whenever such may be suggested by the surveillance data, and also to evaluate the effectiveness of various infection control procedures and policies.
9. To maintain close liaison with the employees health service and to monitor infection in hospital personnel.
10. To review infection data with the hospital epidemiologist.
11. To report specific notifiable infections from all hospital areas to the health authorities.
12. To monitor the environment.
13. To conduct a weekly check and special studies on the adequacy of sterilization procedures for the operating room, central supply, obstetrics, and emergency room.
14. To monitor the techniques utilized by medical and paramedical personnel, such as aseptic techniques, isolation procedures, and disinfection.
15. To monitor antibiotic use—obtain antibiotic lists from the pharmacy.
16. To analyze weekly and monthly the surveillance data on nosocomial infections in regard to specific organisms (weekly), specific wards (weekly), services, physicians, and therapeutic modalities, such as urinary catheters and intermittent positive pressure breathing (monthly).
17. To attend infection control committee meetings.
18. To be responsible for the disposition of patients into and out of isolation. If any problems arise, the NE will refer them to the chairman of the infection control committee and/or the hospital epidemiologist.
19. To consult on placement of patients with infections or patients with increased susceptibility to infection.
20. To supplement control measures when infection problems arise.
21. To be responsible for the education of new personnel and to keep all personnel and physicians abreast of current policies regarding surveillance data. The NE provides these personnel with the analysis of surveillance data as it may pertain to them or their departments.
22. To work with the school of medical technology. Each student will spend one week with the NE as he or she rotates through the bacteriology department. The NE is responsible to see that the students become familiar with the procedures and principles of hospital epidemiology.
23. To attend workshops or seminars as designated by the hospital epidemiologist and/or hospital administration to keep abreast of current methods and trends in hospital epidemiology.
24. To be directly accountable to the hospital epidemiologist.

Although a nurse is often the best person available to meet the qualifications and carry out the responsibilities of this position, many institutions have found other persons such as medical technologists or microbiologists to be equally satisfactory. An effective infection control program cannot result when the position of NE is created and then filled by the lateral move of an incompetent person from another area; unfortunately this is not infrequent.

There is no magic number or ratio for how many NEs per number of patients there should be. The current figure of one NE per 250 patients may serve as a guide, but the number should be determined on an individual institutional basis according to what is needed to accomplish the duties and responsibilities of the position. An extended care facility may require a lower ratio, whereas a primarily intensive care facility probably requires a higher ratio.

HOSPITAL EPIDEMIOLOGIST

The hospital epidemiologist (HE) is the director of the hospital epidemiology program. The qualifications and responsibilities of this position are usually best met by a physician, preferably one based at the hospital. The duties and responsibilities of the HE in our institution include (but are not necessarily limited to) the following:

1. To oversee the entire infection control program.
2. To provide direction, guidance, and support for the NE, particularly in areas of actual or potential conflict with physicians, administration, or other personnel.
3. To review and analyze daily the results of the NE's findings, particularly problem cases and situations.
4. To analyze infection surveillance data.
5. To conduct investigations of outbreaks and other infection problems in the hospital.
6. To analyze data provided by surveillance, audits, and other studies on the use and abuse of antimicrobial agents, indwelling urinary catheters, intravenous cannulae, and other practices.
7. To conduct regular evaluation of the adequacy of isolation procedures, sanitation procedures, sterilization procedures, and the infection reporting system.
8. To carry out the recommendations of the infection control committee as approved by the executive committee.
9. To serve as the liaison between the hospital and local health department.
10. To be directly accountable to the hospital administration and the infection control committee.

The position of HE is rarely a full-time one except, perhaps, in large, acute care hospitals. In most hospitals the job requires only two to ten hours each week. It should include frequent conferences with the NE to discuss in-house problems and to review and analyze surveillance data. Because of the in-house nature of the duties, the responsibilities of the position usually can be filled best by a hospital-based physician (or other qualified person) such as a pathologist who has experience and interest in epidemiology. However, the most qualified and interested person often is a member of the medical staff, such as an internist with a special interest in infectious diseases. In such instances a nonhospital-based physician should be appointed as the hospital epidemiologist, and because of the accountability to hospital administration, that person should be paid for this service.

NURSE EPIDEMIOLOGIST ASSISTANTS

Many of the NE's chores involve paperwork such as data collection in tabular form, statistical analyses, and written communication (both interdepartmental as well as outside the institution). When the work load for an NE becomes too much for one person, it may be more cost-effective to employ someone at a clerical or secretarial level than to hire an additional professional NE. The requirements for such a position are not as great and include interest and educability.

OTHERS

Although the members of the hospital epidemiology department provide the framework for infection control programs, these programs cannot succeed without the support and cooperation of all hospital personnel as well as the medical staff. The hospital administrator must be committed to the concept of an effective infection control program and provide appropriate financial support. All hospital department heads play a role and cooperate with the NE not only in the continuous in-service education of the members of each department but also in executing their own responsibilities. Laboratory personnel, particularly microbiologists, are key resource personnel for the NE, and it is essential that there be close communication and cooperation between these two; they should exploit each other's data and expertise in their daily work. The medical staff plays a critical role not only in understanding and cooperating but also in providing insights and input to the program. There is nothing more disconcerting or damaging to an infection control program than a medical staff member who thinks he or she is an exception to the rules and regulations regarding infection control. By setting an example, the medical staff sets the tone for the success or failure of an infection control program.

SURVEILLANCE

Surveillance refers to the monitoring within the health care facility of infections as well as environmental conditions and hospital practices that may have a bearing on the development of infection. Surveillance is a duty of the NE. It is conveniently divided into three major types: environmental surveillance, infection surveillance, and surveillance of policies, procedures, and personnel practices. A fourth type of surveillance, antibiotic surveillance, may or may not fall into the NE's domain; this depends largely on the medical staff organization.

As stated above, surveillance by itself is meaningless. To have value it must be goal-directed. Questions such as those listed below should be answered satisfactorily before the surveillance is implemented:

1. What is the problem or potential problem to be investigated?
2. What is the goal of the proposed surveillance program?
3. What are the possible results of the surveillance?
4. Are all the possible results interpretable? *a.* Are standards available for comparison? *b.* Are all significant or potentially significant variables included and considered in the surveillance data?
5. Will the surveillance data be used to accomplish the stated goals and purposes of the surveillance program? *a.* Can and will the data be used to support or alter current practices? *b.* Is there a means for effectively altering practices that surveillance data reveal to be "substandard"?

Certainly, if no beneficial effect can be foreseen to result from the surveillance, then there is no justification for it. Too often surveillance programs are initiated because of accreditation requirements or the successes of other hospitals, without understanding the goals of surveillance or the ultimate effect that might result. Such approaches should be discouraged.

ENVIRONMENTAL SURVEILLANCE

Prior to the late 1960s, environmental surveillance was the only form of surveillance practiced by most hospitals—largely because of accreditation requirements. Environmental surveillance was primarily bacteriologic culture monitoring of items such as floors, walls, bedspreads, utensils, and ice. The methods used were usually of unproved value and haphazard at best, and this was reflected in the data accumulated. Standards for acceptable numbers or types of bacteria in the environment were either unavailable or extremely controversial. As a result, hospitals spent considerable amounts of money to accumulate large volumes of data that were usually uninterpretable and from which no course of action could be derived. Aside from epidemic situations, this form of routine environmental surveillance has shown no appreciable correlation with the prevalence of nosocomial infections, and it has not contributed in any significant way to an understanding of the epidemiology or control of nosocomial infection.

There are several specific indications for environmental culture surveillance. Before one institutes any form of culture surveillance, however, the questions listed above should be answered as completely as possible. If these questions can be answered satisfactorily, specific environmental culture plans will have merit. One of the major problems is how to interpret the results—particularly when items with a normal flora are cultured. The results of culturing items that are supposed to be sterile are much easier to interpret. The following are some examples of culture surveillance that have been utilized in an effective way:

1. Epidemic investigations.—In hospital infection outbreaks in which no source is readily apparent, extensive cultures taken from environmental items and personnel may detect the source of the outbreak, thus providing the information necessary to establish effective measures to end the outbreak and prevent future recurrences.

2. Equipment monitoring.—This includes periodic cultures taken from specific items, eg, respiratory therapy equipment. Respiratory therapy equipment has been incriminated as the cause of a number. of nosocomial respiratory infection outbreaks; the cause is often traced to a reservoir of the infectious agent in a humidifier or nebulizer. Periodic spot checking by cultures taken from reusable tubing, humidifiers, and nebulizers can be useful in detecting problems or potential problems early, thus providing justification for quick remedial or prophylactic measures.

3. Education.—Sometimes environmental cultures may be useful in the in-service educational programs by the NE. For example, cultures taken from items before and after proper and improper cleaning or disinfection procedures may be most useful in dramatizing the importance of certain procedures.

Environmental surveillance, however, must not be looked upon as primarily culture surveillance. In fact, today culture surveillance constitutes a relatively small component of environmental surveillance. Some of the more important aspects of environmental surveillance are given below.

Visual Inspection.—Environmental surveillance should include visual inspection of the entire hospital on a routine basis—from the operating room to the nursing units, from central supply to purchasing, from administration to the dietary department. Is the environment clean on visual inspection? There should be a quality control mechanism for the housekeeping department, which should logically include the NE's input in its design and operation. It should include means of answering the following questions: Are all areas and articles cleaned at appropriate intervals?

Are appropriate disinfectants being used? Are they reconstituted to the recommended dilutions? Many areas in the hospital require special and/or increased housekeeping attention (eg, operating rooms, ICUs, and kitchens). Requirements must be specifically spelled out and included in the quality control checks.

Antiseptics and Disinfectants Surveillance. — The NE must become familiar with acceptable disinfecting compounds and their proper use and application. Are approved agents being used in areas and in circumstances for which they are approved? This must be checked on a regular basis because new agents have a way of creeping into use without going through an appropriate approval process. Many hospitals have a new product evaluation committee that evaluates new products proposed for routine use in the hospital. The NE should be a member of this committee or at least be a consultant when products such as soaps, disinfectants, and antiseptics are being considered. This means that the NE must be familiar with the evaluation procedures of such agents and the interpretations of the results. In-house testing of the efficacy of such products should not be considered a part of such an evaluation and should not be performed normally. The evaluation should include questions such as: Has the agent been approved by appropriate certifying agencies such as the US Food and Drug Administration? How has it been tested and how do the results compare with those of agents in current use? What are the advantages and disadvantages of the proposed agent/compound in relation to that being used currently? What comparable institution uses the proposed product and who can be contacted there for an in-use evaluation report? Many acceptable agents are available for various uses. Table 8-1 lists some examples of the more common products and their uses. This should not be considered an all-inclusive list.

Autoclave Sterilization Check. — Autoclaves, either steam or ethylene oxide, are used when the final products must be absolutely sterile, eg, for surgical instruments. It is therefore essential that the autoclave function properly, and this can be assured only by appropriate monitoring, which should take at least two forms. There should be regular monitoring (daily, weekly, or monthly depending on frequency of use) of the sporicidal activity of each autoclave. Preparations of spores of *Bacillus stearothermophilis* (steam autoclave) and *B subtilis* (gas autoclave) are commercially available. In addition, each use of the autoclave should be checked to assure that an appropriate critical (minimum) temperature is attained and maintained for at least the minimum accepted time. A convenient but not totally reliable method is the use of temperature-sensitive indicator tape, which can be applied to the outside of autoclaved packages. This does not prove that appropriate conditions were obtained in the center of the package, however.

Autoclaves that have demonstrated incompetence must be removed from service until repaired. Records of test results and maintenance of autoclaves should be kept.

TABLE 8-1.—Examples of Acceptable Means of Sterilization, Disinfection, and Antisepsis

USES	ACCEPTABLE AGENTS	RESULT*
Objects (inanimate) without tissue, mucosal, or significant skin contact	Alcohol, 70%-90% (ethyl or isopropyl)	D
	Hypochlorite	D
	Iodophors (100 ppm available I_2)	D
	Phenols	D
	Quaternary ammonium compounds, 2% aqueous	D
Rubber and plastic objects with skin or mucosal contact	Ethylene oxide	S
	Glutaraldehyde, 2%	D, S
	Iodophors (500 ppm available I_2)	D
	Steam, autoclave	S
Endoscopes	Ethylene oxide	S
	Formaldehyde	D, S
	Glutaraldehyde	D, S
Tissue or intravascular instruments or catheters	Ethylene oxide	S
	Steam autoclave	S
Cutaneous antiseptics	Iodophors	A
	Iodine, 0.2% in 70% alcohol	A
	Chlorhexidine	A
	Hexachlorophene	A

*Abbreviations: A, antisepsis; D, disinfection; S, sterilization.

Food.—The dietary department provides a particularly difficult challenge to environmental surveillance. The major problem is the unavailability of acceptable standards. The hospital food service department is required to meet specifications no more stringent than those required for restaurants that serve the general public, yet hospital kitchens are preparing food for ill patients who have decreased resistance to infections.

Furthermore, microbes that cause infections are being traced increasingly to food and/or the hospital kitchen.[94, 275] In the absence of acceptable standards, it is not practical to recommend stringent surveillance measures. At present, one can recommend that NEs visit the kitchen regularly and frequently, thereby making their presence and concern known to the food service personnel; observe the general cleanliness; and perhaps go through a general checklist of questions such as: Is food being left out at room temperature? Are refrigerator and freezer temperatures adequate? Does the dishwasher water attain appropriately high temperatures?

INFECTION SURVEILLANCE

Infection surveillance refers to the monitoring of all hospitalized patients for the presence of infections and the development of nosocomial infections. It would be impossible for the NE to check each patient daily for infection. There are a number of much more productive and less time-consuming means of infection detection, including those listed below.

1. Microbiology culture log.—For most surveillance systems the microbiology laboratory constitutes the single most fruitful source of information on infected patients. One can assume that any patient from whom a culture has been taken is one in whom there is at least a clinical suspicion of infection. Consequently, any patient listed in the microbiology log should be checked by the NE. Those with negative cultures should be checked for other possible infections, eg, viral infections or infections at other sites.

2. Daily admission list.—The admitting department usually can supply the NE with a daily list of all new admissions and their admitting diagnoses. Some patients are admitted with diagnoses of infection, which simplifies their detection. Other patients are admitted with diagnoses of diseases that are particularly vulnerable to infection, eg, diabetes, leukemia, and lymphoma. The list provides the NE with the names of those patients who must be checked more carefully during routine ward rounds for evidence of infection.

3. Other laboratory data lists.—There are many laboratory tests outside the microbiology section with results that may strongly suggest the presence of infection. Examples include elevated white blood cell counts with an increased percentage of neutrophil band cells, marked leukopenia, atypical lymphocytes in the peripheral blood smear, markedly elevated serum transaminase levels, and bacteriuria. A system whereby such abnormal results are routinely reported to the NE is desirable. This is implemented easily if the laboratory utilizes a computer but may be impractical otherwise.

4. **X-ray lists.**—Routine review of all chest x-ray diagnoses made by the radiology department can provide the NE with a list of patients with high likelihood of having respiratory tract infections.
5. **Antibiotic list.**—Patients who are receiving antibiotics can be presumed to have a known or suspected infection, or they may be receiving them prophylactically. A daily list of such patients provided by the pharmacy department can be most helpful to the NE in finding cases of infection.
6. **Autopsies.**—Autopsy reports should be reviewed on a regular basis for evidence of infection not detected antemortem.

The most critical and effective method available to the NE for finding infections in the hospital is routine ward rounds. It is not necessary to evaluate every patient individually on such rounds—in fact, to do so is relatively ineffective. The NE should prepare a list of patients with high likelihood or possibility of infection—a list derived from one or more of the sources mentioned above. The patients on this list should be evaluated carefully by the NE for the presence or absence of infection, based on consistent criteria such as those listed in Table 1-1. During ward rounds the NE should also discuss with the nursing supervisor of each unit the patients who do have or may have infections. Also, the unit supervisors are invaluable sources of information about other patients who may have infections, eg, patients with unexplained fevers. Close communication and good rapport between the NE and all unit supervisors are perhaps the best assurances of the most complete and accurate detection of infections in the hospital.

Once an infection is diagnosed, the NE must categorize it as being either community-acquired or nosocomial, again utilizing rigid consistent criteria such as those listed in Table 1-2. Most hospital epidemiology programs currently do not keep close tabs on community-acquired infections, which may be a mistake. The NE constantly should be aware of what is occurring in the community in relation to infection. There should be a close relationship between the NE and local health departments. Many infections are required by law to be reported to the health department. The NE can provide a valuable service to the community by being aware of and keeping track of the cases of community-acquired infections admitted to the hospital and reporting to the health department not only those required by law but also any other infections or clusters of infections that might suggest an epidemic or problem. In addition, the NE should be aware of community-acquired infections in order to initiate any precautions that may be necessary to prevent the transmission of the infection to other patients or personnel.

Epidemiologic Data.—When a nosocomial infection has been identified, epidemiologic data on the patient(s) involved should be obtained by the NE. These should include information on the items listed in Table 8-2. Depending on the experience and goals of the NE, such a list can be short-

TABLE 8-2.—Epidemiologic Data Helpful
in Monitoring Nosocomial Infections

Date of admission
Date of infection onset
Site of infection
Etiologic agent of infection
Location of patient in hospital
Specialty service, if any
Urinary catheters, if any
Intravenous catheters, if any
Respiratory therapy, if any
Anesthesia, if any
Surgical procedure, if any
Physicians
Age and sex of patient
Underlying primary diseases
Antibiotics used before onset of infection
Immunosuppressant agents, if any

---

ened or expanded. There is little justification, however, for collecting data for which one foresees no possible utilization.

The data must be stored in an easily retrievable fashion. This can be done conveniently on a computer, but a computer is not available to most NEs. A line-listing format and various card systems have proved reliable.

Data Tabulation.—At regular intervals the data must be tabulated and displayed in a system that is easy to understand. From an epidemiologic standpoint, there are at least three major factors that should be included in such analytic displays: site of infection, infecting agent, and location or service of patient. To display simply, the interrelationships among the three factors require the following three tables: (1) number of infections by site of infection in each nursing unit or service (Table 8-3); (2) number of infections by infecting agent in each nursing unit or service (Table 8-4); and (3) frequency of infecting agent and infection site (Table 8-5). Such displays should be prepared at least monthly, but for larger institutions, it may be more effective to prepare them weekly.

After data have been accumulated for one to two years, there should be sufficient data to calculate endemic nosocomial infection rates. For example, one can calculate the mean monthly urinary tract infection rate for each

TABLE 8-3.—Distribution of Nosocomial Infections in Nursing Unit
(St. Vincent Hospital and Medical Center)

Month October, 1978

UNIT	WD	RTI	UTI	BACTEREMIA	IVC	MISC.	TOTAL
NBN							0
OB							0
A	1					1	2
B		1	2				3
C							0
D	2	2	5			1	10
E	1		1				2
F	1	2	2				5
G		4*	2	1		2	9
H	2 (1)		2	(1)		1	5 (1)
I	2	1	2				5
J	1	1	1				3
K	1		2				3
CRR	1		1	(1)	1 (1)		3 (1)
ICU	1	1	4 (1)	1 (1)		1	8 (1)
Totals	13 (1)	12	24 (1)	2 (3)	1 (1)	6	58 (3)

*1977 mean = 0.83; 2SD = 1.99.
Abbreviations: CRR, cardiac recovery room; ICU, intensive care unit; IVC, intravenous catheter infections; NBN, newborn nursery; OB, obstetrics; RTI, respiratory tract infections; UTI, urinary tract infections; WD, wound infections.
Number in parentheses ( ) = 2° bacteremias.

nursing unit and for the hospital as a whole. The standard deviation can then be calculated. A figure of twice the standard deviation (2 SD) indicates the variation in the current endemic infection rate 95% of the time. Infection rate values greater than the 2 SD figure should be considered unusual and merit investigation. The means and 2 SD figures should be calculated annually for each of the data tables. Table 8-6 is an example. The NE then can compare each month the current monthly infection rates

Hospital-Associated Infections

TABLE 8–4.—Prevalent Microbe Distribution in Nursing Unit
(St. Vincent Hospital and Medical Center)

Month   October, 1978

	E coli	S aureus	K pneumoniae	C albicans	S faecalis	P aeruginosa	P mirabilis	B fragilis	S marcescens	S epidermidis
NBN										
OB										
A	1				1					
B	1		1				1			
C										
D	3	1	1	1	1		2	1		1
E	1	1								
F	2		1				1		1	
G	1	1	5*			1			1	2
H	2 (1)	1		1	1			1		
I	3		1							
J	1	1								1
K	2	1			1					
CRR		1 (1)	1						1	
ICU	1		2	1		2 (1)			1	1
Totals	18 (1)	7 (1)	12	3	4	3 (1)	4	2	4	5

*1977 mean = 0.75; 2SD = 2.48.

Abbreviations: CRR, cardiac recovery room; ICU, intensive care unit; IVC, intravenous catheter infections; NBN, newborn nursery; OB, obstetrics; RTI, respiratory tract infections; UTI, urinary tract infections; WD, wound infections.

Number in parentheses ( ) = 2° bacteremias.

TABLE 8-5.—Nosocomial Microbe and Site Frequency
(St. Vincent Hospital and Medical Center)

Month   October, 1978

	WD	BLOOD	LRT	UTI	MISC.	TOTALS
Acinetobacter calcoaceticus					1	1
Bacillus species						
Bacteroides fragilis	2					2
Candida albicans			1	2		3
Candida tropicalis						
Clostridium perfringens	1					1
Corynebacterium species						
Diplococcus pneumoniae			1			1
Enterobacter aerogenes				1		1
Enterobacter cloacae			1			1
Enterobacter agglomerans						
Escherichia coli	4 (1)	1 (1)		13		18 (1)
Hemophilus influenzae						
Hemophilus parainfluenzae						
Hemophilus vaginalis						
Klebsiella pneumoniae*	1		6*	4	1	12
Peptostreptococcus species	1					1
Proteus mirabilis				4		4
Proteus morgani						
Pseudomonas aeruginosa	2	(1)		1 (1)		3 (1)
Serratia marcescens	1		2		1	4
Staphylococcus aureus	3	1 (1)	1		2 (1)	7 (1)
Staphylococcus epidermidis	2			2	1	5
Streptococcus pyogenes (A)						
Streptococcus agalactiae (B)						
Streptococcus (NGABD)(β)						
Streptococcus (NGABD)(γ)						
Streptococcus durans						
Streptococcus faecium						
Streptococcus faecalis	2			1	1	4
Streptococcus liquefaciens						
Streptococcus viridans						
Torulopsis glabrata						

*There was a significantly increased incidence of *K pneumoniae* RTIs in unit G. Biotypes of four isolates were identical. Possible common source. Investigation under way.

TABLE 8-6.—Means and Standard Deviations of Nosocomial Infections
(St. Vincent Hospital and Medical Center, 1977)

	WOUNDS		RESPIRATORY TRACT		URINARY TRACT		MISCELLANEOUS		TOTAL	
	Mean	2SD	Mean	2SD	Mean	2SD	Mean	2SD	Mean	2SD
NB	0.08	0.66	0	0	0	0	0.42	1.75	0.50	2.31
OB	0.33	1.64	0.17	0.95	0.67	2.64	0.08	0.66	1.25	4.57
A	0.33	1.32	0.75	2.68	0.42	1.45	0.33	1.64	1.83	4.22
B	0.50	1.85	0.75	3.59	1.83	4.89	0.17	0.95	3.25	7.08
C	0.08	0.66	0.42	1.75	0.75	1.99	0.08	0.66	1.33	3.64
D	1.08	3.08	0.67	2.64	5.00	10.33	0.33	1.32	7.08	13.98
E	0.17	1.32	0.50	1.85	1.83	4.51	0.25	1.15	2.75	6.07
F	0.17	0.95	1.75	5.28	2.50	4.67	1.00	3.09	5.42	10.12
G	0.08	0.66	0.83	1.99	2.58	5.06	0.50	2.10	4.00	7.52
H	1.58	3.75	1.17	4.10	2.83	6.82	0.42	2.00	6.00	11.33
I	2.33	5.88	0.83	3.22	2.92	5.93	0.75	2.68	6.83	13.43
J	0.33	1.32	0.58	1.92	1.92	4.25	0.33	1.64	3.17	6.96
K	0.25	1.15	0.33	1.32	2.42	5.98	0	0	3.00	6.30
CRR	0.58	2.17	0.67	2.81	0.75	2.68	0.58	2.38	2.58	5.83
ICU	0.25	1.49	3.08	6.33	2.42	5.55	1.08	3.25	6.83	12.35
Totals	8.17	13.81	12.50	22.43	28.92	48.03	6.33	9.88	55.83	75.15

with the mean and standard deviation values of the previous year. If the infection rates fall within the 2 SD range, there is probably no outbreak problem, but any figure exceeding the 2 SD value must be explained or investigated.

Employee Infection Surveillance. — Infection surveillance is not limited to patients. Not only are hospital personnel susceptible to many infections, but when infected, they may be a source of infections for patients. Consequently, it is important for the NE to be aware of personnel infections throughout the hospital. The NE should try to determine whether an infection was acquired in the hospital and whether there are risks of transmission to others. This requires close communication and cooperation with the hospital's employee health service.

Outbreak Investigation. — One final activity that falls best under the heading of infection surveillance is the investigation of outbreaks. When an outbreak is detected or suspected, a fairly simple protocol can be followed to aid in determining whether there is a true outbreak, and if so, what are the most productive avenues of further investigations. Although there are many variations on this protocol, certain basic concepts are common to most of them. These include the following:

1. Case definition.—A careful description with measurable objective criteria must be selected for cases in the epidemic.
2. Control group.—One or more control populations must be selected that are as similar as possible to the cases.
3. Chart review.—A list of all conceivable epidemiologic factors is made for both cases and controls, and these are then compared.

The following case can serve as an example. During one August there were six cases of nosocomial UTI due to *Serratia marcescens* in unit X. The monthly mean and 2SD for UTIs and for *S marcescens* infections in this unit were 2.1 ± 2.7 and 0.8 ± 1.5, respectively. The figures for August clearly suggested an outbreak. There were no other *S marcescens* UTIs in August in the rest of the hospital. The following procedure was followed:

1. The case definition used was: All nosocomial *S marcescens* UTIs in unit X occurring after August 1.
2. Two control populations were selected:
    a. All nosocomial *S marcescens* UTIs occurring in unit X during the 12 months prior to August 1.
    b. Every tenth patient admitted to unit X during August who did not develop a *S marcescens* UTI.
3. By chart review, the following epidemiologic factors were collected and compared: age, sex, infection date, interval between admission and infection, room number, service, physician, urinary catheter, who

inserted catheter, infecting organism—biotype, underlying disease, immunosuppressant therapy, and surgery.

Unit X is primarily a medical oncology unit. Most patients in both groups were oncology patients, and hence this category (service) is omitted from Table 8-7. Table 8-7 lists the distribution of the above factors in the cases and controls. An additional case that occurred in early September also is included.

It is clear from examining the data in Tables 8-7 and 8-8 that: (1) an outbreak in unit X has indeed occurred, (2) cases are significantly related to urinary catheterization, and (3) there is a strong suggestion of relationship to person N, one of three people responsible for inserting catheters into patients in unit X. The data from this brief review nicely points out the direction for further investigation. Cultures of hands, nose, throat, and anal swabs were obtained from all personnel including N, and all were negative for *S marcescens*. Careful review and observation of the techniques used for catheter insertion revealed the following: The standard policy for cleaning the perineum and perineal area required the use of povidone-iodine provided with each catheter set. N thought she might be allergic to iodine and in mid-summer began to use a green soap solution she prepared herself and kept in the utility room. A culture of the solution grew numerous gram-negative organisms, including *S marcescens*. Once this was brought to light, N returned to using standard cleaning procedures and the outbreak ceased.

Most nosocomial outbreaks are not explained so easily and often require much improvisation and initiative on the part of the investigator. The most common causes for failure are: (1) poor case definitions, (2) inadequate control groups, and (3) failure to ask the right epidemiologic questions on chart review.

SURVEILLANCE OF POLICIES, PROCEDURES, AND PRACTICES

This surveillance involves the monitoring of all hospital policies and procedures that may have any bearing on the development or control of infections, and also monitoring of all practices to determine whether they conform to hospital policies and procedures. This form of surveillance often is assumed to be implicit in environmental and infection surveillance. Although admittedly there is some overlap, the importance of such monitoring and its frequent neglect justify explicit consideration.

Since there is virtually no hospital department or service that lacks direct or indirect contact with patients, the problem of potential infection transmission exists for them all—although the risks vary considerably among them. Each department or service should have a set of procedures and policies specific for its particular area, and all personnel should be

TABLE 8-7.—Epidemiologic Parameters in *S marcescens* Urinary Tract Infection Outbreak in Unit X

CASE NO.	AGE	SEX	INFECTION DATE	INTERVAL SINCE ADMISSION (DAYS)	ROOM	PHYS.	CATHETER	INSERTED BY	DISEASE	IMMUNO-SUPPRESSANT THERAPY	ORGANISM*/BIOTYPE
Cases											
1	56	F	8/7	4	X23	A	Yes	N	HD	Yes	SM/4
2	63	F	8/12	6	X33	B	Yes	N	AML	Yes	SM/4
3	66	F	8/12	7	X45	C	Yes	N	Lymphoma	Yes	SM/4
4	72	M	8/15	3	X19	B	Yes	N	Lymphoma	Yes	SM/4
5	60	F	8/22	8	X24	D	Yes	P	Breast Cancer	No	SM/4
6	6	M	8/30	10	X29	C	Yes	N	ALL	Yes	SM/4
7	59	F	9/30	5	X33	B	Yes	N	PCM	Yes	SM/4
Control group #1											
1	58	F	1/16	8	X24	B	Yes	P	Breast Cancer	Yes	SM/1
2	74	F	5/14	5	X20	D	Yes	R	Lymphoma	Yes	SM/4
Control group #2											
1	65	M			X20	B	No		Lymphoma	No	
2	62	M			X42	B	No		Aplast. anemia	Yes	
3	71	F			X44	D	Yes	N	Lung Cancer	Yes	
4	66	F			X28	A	No		Breast Cancer	Yes	
5	54	F	8/16	6	X21	C	Yes	R	AML	Yes	EC/18
6	88	M			X34	C	No		PCM	Yes	
7	71	F			X23	B	No		Lymphoma	Yes	
8	45	M			X29	E	No		HD	Yes	
9	60	F			X34	B	Yes	P	Breast Cancer	Yes	

*Organisms: SM, *Serratia marcescens*; EC, *Escherichia coli.*

TABLE 8-8.—Summary of Pertinent Epidemiologic Data from Table 8-7

GROUP	AGE MEAN RANGE	SEX (F/M)	RATIO	ROOM	PHYSICIAN	CATHETER	INSERTED BY	IMMUNO-SUPPRESSANT THERAPY	ORGANISM/BIOTYPE
Cases (7)	55 6-72	5/2	0.71	X33 twice, Others once	A-1, B-3, C-2, D-1,	Yes-100%	N-86% P-14%	Yes-86%	SM/4-100%
Control #1 (2)	61 58-74	2/0	1.00	Both different	B-1, D-1,	Yes-100%	P-50% R-50%	Yes-100%	SM/4-50%
Control #2 (9)	65 45-88	5/4	0.55	X34 twice, Others once	A-1, B-4, C-2, D-1, E-1,	Yes-33%	N-33% P-33% R-33%	Yes-89%	SM/4-0 EC/18-1

familiar with these as well as with those common to the hospital as a whole. Ideally, each department should have a manual that describes the infection control policies and procedures of the hospital in general and the specific department in particular. The NE should have a master manual that includes the policies and procedures of all departments and services as well as those of the overall hospital. The policies and procedures and any subsequent changes should be approved by the infection control committee.

The initial surveillance of current hospital policies and procedures is often a most eye-opening experience. There are often different policies and procedures in different nursing units for carrying out the same order, or there may be no policy at all. For example, initial surveillance in our hospital revealed urinary catheter care policies in only two nursing units, and these differed considerably; the remaining units had no policy at all. Such data provide abundant material for analysis and corrective action.

Policies and procedures are meaningless unless they are carried out. In the example cited above, no significant reduction occurred in the rate of nosocomial urinary tract infection following institution of a uniform catheter care policy until a year later, when steps were taken to assure execution of the new policy and procedures (Fig 8-1). It is thus important for NEs to monitor infection control practices as part of their surveillance duties. This is often easily done by observation during regular rounds and by casual interviews of personnel in various departments.

Once hospital policies and procedures are established, they must not be considered sacrosanct or unchangeable. The NE must be aware of new and more effective procedures and techniques as they become available and initiate the steps needed to introduce the proved procedures into the hospital.

ANTIBIOTIC SURVEILLANCE

There is no more controversial or emotionally charged type of surveillance than that of the use of antimicrobial agents. Surveillance alone, however, has no value; it must have a purpose. The data must be collected and analyzed with the ultimate goal of utilizing them in a rational way to increase the appropriate use of antimicrobics. The problem is defining the appropriate use of antimicrobics.

There is general consensus that antimicrobial agents are greatly overused and misused.[319] On the other hand, it has not been possible to reach a consensus on where to draw the line between appropriate and inappropriate use. Nevertheless, most hospitals are required to have some form of antibiotic use auditing by accrediting agencies such as the Joint Commission on Accreditation of Hospitals. This is a true dilemma facing hospitals today. They are required to conduct antibiotic use audits without any

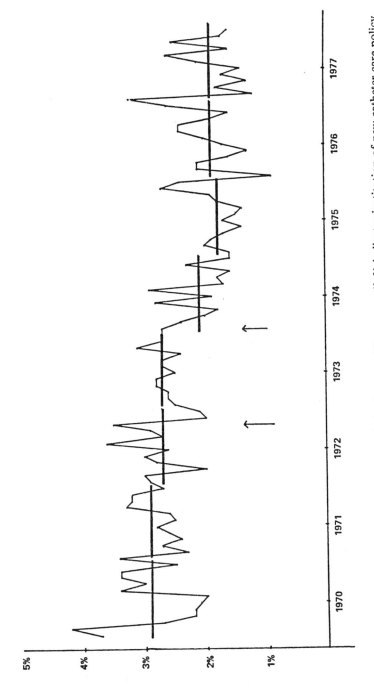

Fig 8–1. Overall monthly urinary tract infection rate. First arrow (*left*) indicates institution of new catheter care policy. Second arrow (*right*) indicates institution of intensive in-service education and surveillance of catheter care practice. Dark horizontal lines are annual means. (St. Vincent Hospital and Medical Center, 1970–1977.)

guidelines and with no guarantee that the results will effectively alter (let alone improve) the antimicrobic prescribing practices of physicians. A few studies have shown that requiring physician justification for the use of certain antibiotics (eg, aminoglycosides) has reduced their use.[133, 392] In the absence of hard data to serve as models or guidelines, it is important to embark on such surveillance with considerable forethought. The principles of surveillance in general and the questions regarding the goals and ability to accomplish these goals must be studied carefully. Particularly important in antibiotic surveillance is the selection of standards and the planned means of modifying the practice of those whose use of antibiotics is considered substandard in some way.

Although experience in this area is limited, we make the following suggestion: if surveillance data can be collected and presented to the medical staff in such a way that the use of specific antimicrobics in a particular situation is clearly superior or inferior to another practice, the majority of physicians undoubtedly will draw the appropriate conclusions and quite voluntarily make appropriate changes in their practice. In order to accomplish this, it is necessary to select highly specific problems, eg, the use of prophylactic antimicrobics in bowel surgery. One can conduct intense surveillance of infections and practices (including use of prophylactic antimicrobics) on all patients who have bowel surgery. After a specified period of time or a certain number of cases, the data can be analyzed to determine whether there is any correlation between prophylactic antibiotic use and postoperative wound infection rates. If a particular practice clearly stands out as superior or inferior to others, appropriate presentation of such data to the medical staff will certainly have an effect on future practice. In such a context, the medical staff can determine for itself what its standards should be—based on the members' own collective experiences.

Surveillance of the therapeutic use of antimicrobics can be accomplished similarly. For example, what is the antibiotic practice in treating patients with suspected gram-negative pneumonia before the diagnosis is established? How does the response to therapy correlate with the antibiotic used? Is there a difference in duration of hospital stay? If such correlations are found and presented appropriately to the medical staff, corresponding changes in practice certainly will follow.

To attempt to achieve 100% uniformity of practice in the use of antimicrobics (as well as any other medical practice) is clearly undesirable for the following reasons: (1) Despite the unquestioned superiority of certain drugs for treating certain conditions, eg, penicillin G for pneumococcal pneumonia, extenuating circumstances are often sufficient to justify (or even demand) the use of an alternative drug (eg, cases of penicillin hypersensitivity). (2) Complete uniformity of practice stifles progress, since it prevents the introduction of innovations in therapy that should be compared (by surveillance) with current standards and either accepted or rejected based on the results. Antimicrobic surveillance, when conducted in the manner prescribed here, can be informative and may provide clinicians with a basis for rational antimicrobic use.

INFECTION CONTROL COMMITTEE

The infection control committee (ICC) is the central nervous system of the infection control and epidemiology program. The surveillance systems described above correspond to sensory nerves sending information to the central nervous system. The ICC, therefore, is then responsible for interpreting the surveillance data and analyzing them in relation to past experience, current practices, and the experiences and practices of others. Based on such analyses of surveillance information, the ICC is then obliged to implement appropriate control measures whenever indicated. Control measures are usually set up as policies and practices of hospital personnel. Many policies and procedures, however, result in action only when stimulated by specific surveillance data; eg, detection of salmonellosis leads to enteric isolation of the patient. Here the sensory and effector mechanisms act like a reflex; the surveillance (sensory) information does not have to reach the conscious level (ICC) to bring about a control response. It has been previously conditioned by the ICC to react automatically (reflexly) in a specified manner when specific surveillance information is encountered.

Although the ICC is often a medical staff committee, its membership should not be limited to the medical staff but should include certain hospital personnel. The exact composition of the ICC will vary considerably from hospital to hospital depending on the size and nature of the institution. The following may serve as reasonable guidelines:

Medical staff membership should include an expert in infectious diseases as well as at least one representative from each of the major medical staff departments or services. The hospital epidemiologist should also be a member. Hospital personnel membership should include the NE, a microbiologist, and representatives from all the major departments or services directly or indirectly involved with patient care, eg, nursing service, admitting department, housekeeping, and central supply. Membership selections should be made carefully so that people with interest and expertise are chosen in order to ensure efficient and responsible functioning of the committee. Too large and cumbersome a committee should be avoided. Often one person may be a good representative for two or more disciplines that require representation. Ad hoc members from many disciplines may be satisfactory.

The ICC's activities extend far beyond those of the medical staff. Its authority should be sufficient to do whatever is necessary to control the spread of infection in the hospital, eg, to impose isolation when necessary and to close wards if the need is indicated. Such authority cannot be derived from the medical staff and must come from the hospital administration. Consequently, many feel that the ICC should be a hospital committee or at least a joint medical staff–hospital committee. The latter is perhaps a good compromise. In any case, the authority of the ICC must be clearly affirmed. The authority granted must be sufficient to carry out the ICC's responsibilities: to develop and implement measures designed to reduce the nosocomial infection rate to the minimum possible and to prevent the dissemination of extant infections to other patients or personnel. The composition and functions of the ICC at St. Vincent Hospital and Medical Center are as follows:

1. The committee meets monthly and upon indication.
2. Membership includes representation from the following departments:

Administration
Internal medicine, MD
Pathology, MD
Nursing service—administrative,
   staff nurse, operating room nurse
Obstetrics-gynecology, MD
Pediatrics, MD
Surgery, MD

Central supply, RN
Pharmacy
Hospital epidemiologist
Nurse epidemiologist
Infectious disease
   specialist, MD
Admitting department

There is ad hoc participation by representatives of all other departments on a consultative basis.
3. Authority to carry out the functions listed below has been granted by the hospital governing board.
4. Functions include:
   a. To evaluate infections in patients and personnel.
   b. To make recommendations and take appropriate measures to limit further spread from identified sources of contagion.
   c. To ensure adequate isolation policies and procedures.
   d. To report findings and recommendations to the executive committee of the medical staff and the hospital administrator.
   e. To prepare and distribute to the hospital staff regular reports that are pertinent to infection control, eg, antibiotic sensitivity patterns and yearly wound infection rates for individual physicians.
   f. To make certain that all personnel are instructed in the proper practice of medical and surgical asepsis and in their responsibilities in the prevention and control of nosocomial infections.

g. To provide counsel and advice to medical staff and hospital personnel on infection control.

h. To analyze data on infections, evaluate current trends and experience, and undertake such control measures as may be indicated.

i. To monitor antibiotic use.

j. To review practices and procedures that tend to compromise patients' resistance to infection, eg, chemoprophylaxis, immunosuppression by drugs, instrumentation, intubation, and catheterization.

k. To conduct infection prevalence studies to spot check the adequacy of surveillance and infection reporting.

l. To review and update the infection control program at least annually.

m. To review the following items at the monthly meeting (using number of patients discharged as the denominator): number and incidence of nosocomial infections; types of infections; service of infected patients; distribution of nosocomial infections—ward versus site; prevalent microbe distribution—ward versus organism; and nosocomial microbes—site frequency.

CONTROL MEASURES

Like surveillance, control measures should be rational and purposeful. They should be designed to carry out the duties mentioned above in response to or anticipation of actual or potential infection problems in the hospital. The control activities of the ICC may be divided into two categories: immediate and procedural.

IMMEDIATE CONTROL MEASURES

Immediate control measures are those that are set into action immediately in response to specific occurrences. Policies and procedures previously developed by the ICC are designed to permit a quick reaction to the presence of actual or potential hazardous situations. The classical examples are isolation policies and procedures for contagious infections.

Isolation.—Isolation policies, procedures, and practices recommended by the American Hospital Assocation, the Center for Disease Control, and other organizations are readily available and the reader is referred to these sources for details. A brief summary of the types of isolation commonly practiced is given in Table 8-9, and Table 8-10 lists the commonly encountered infections for which isolation is recommended and the corresponding type usually recommended. The following are the isolation policy and procedures at St. Vincent Hospital and Medical Center.

TABLE 8-9.—Types of Isolation

A. *Infection isolation.*—The segregation of patients suffering from contagious infections and the practice of techniques and procedures that prevent the transmission of such infections to other patients and personnel.

  1. *Strict isolation.*—Practice of techniques designed to prevent the transmission of the most contagious infections in which direct contact, fomites, and air are recognized means of communicability.
    a. Private room with running water.
    b. Hand-washing by persons entering and leaving the room.
    c. Gowns worn by persons entering the room and discarded on leaving the room (masks optional).
    d. Special care of linens, dishes, utensils, food, etc.

  2. *Skin and wound isolation.*—Practice of techniques designed to prevent the transmission of infections dependent on contact for their communicability.
    a. Room with running water (private room desirable).
    b. Hand-washing by persons having direct contact with patient—before and after.
    c. Gowns worn by persons having direct contact with patient or bedding.
    d. Gloves worn by persons changing dressings or having other hand contact with infected area.

  3. *Enteric isolation.*—Practice of techniques designed to prevent the transmission of infections dependent on the fecal-oral route for their communicability.
    a. Room with bathroom (private room desirable).
    b. Hand-washing by persons having contact with patient—before and after.
    c. Gowns worn by persons having contact with patient.
    d. Gloves worn by persons having contact with articles with obvious fecal contamination.
    e. "Needle" precautions for patients with hepatitis.

  4. *Respiratory isolation.*—Practice of techniques designed to prevent the transmission of infections dependent on respiratory aerosols for their communicability.
    a. Private room with running water and negative air pressure.
    b. Instruction of patient in sanitary cough techniques.
    c. Gowns (masks optional) for persons attending patients unable to utilize sanitary cough procedures.

B. *Protective isolation (reverse isolation).*—The segregation of patients with extensive increased susceptibility to infections with the practice of techniques designed to minimize exposure of the patient to exogenous microbes.

  1. Private room with running water and positive air pressure.
  2. Sterile gowns, caps, and masks for persons entering room.
  3. Sterile gloves for persons having contact with the patient.
  4. Thorough hand-washing before entering and leaving the room.

TABLE 8-10.—Infections and Suggested Type of Isolation

INFECTION	TYPE OF ISOLATION RECOMMENDED
Anthrax, pulmonary	Strict
Burns with purulent infection	Skin and wound
Cholera	Enteric
Diarrhea, infectious	Enteric
Diphtheria	Strict
Dysentery	Enteric
Gastroenteritis	Enteric
Hepatitis, viral	Enteric with needle precautions
Herpes simplex, labialis	None
Herpes simplex, disseminated	Strict
Herpes zoster, localized	Skin and wound
Impetigo	Strict
Influenza	None
Measles	Respiratory
Meningitis, nonmeningococcal	None
Meningococcal disease	Respiratory
Mumps	Respiratory
Mycoses, systemic	None
Pertussis	Respiratory
Plague, pneumonic	Strict
Pneumonia, pneumococcal	None
Pneumonia, staphylococcal	Strict
Rabies	Strict
Rickettsial infections	None
Rubella	Respiratory
Skin or wound infection, purulent, draining, staphylococcal	Strict
Skin or wound infection, purulent, draining, other	Skin and wound
Tuberculosis, pulmonary	Respiratory
Typhoid	Enteric
Urinary tract infection	None
Vaccinia, generalized	Strict
Varicella and disseminated zoster	Strict

ISOLATION POLICY

I. Definition of isolation.

A. Source isolation is the segregation of patients suffering from contagious infectious diseases and the practice of medical asepsis for the purpose of preventing the transmission of such diseases to other patients and personnel. Based on the degree and mechanism of contagion, four types of source isolation are practiced.

    1. Enteric isolation is the practice of techniques (see below) designed to prevent the transmission of infections dependent on the fecal-oral route for their communicability.

    2. Skin and wound isolation is the practice of techniques (see below) designed to prevent the transmission of infections dependent on direct person-to-person contact for their communicability.

    3. Strict isolation is the practice of techniques (see below) designed to prevent the transmission of the most contagious infections in which direct contact, fomites, and air are recognized means of communicability.

    4. Respiratory isolation is the practice of techniques (see below) designed to prevent the transmission of infections primarily spread by droplets or aerosols resulting from coughing or sneezing.

B. Protective isolation is the segregation of patients with increased susceptibility to infections and the practice of aseptic techniques designed to minimize exposure of such patients to exogenous microbes.

II. Aims.

The primary purpose of this isolation policy is to provide guidelines and regulations to prevent transmission of infectious diseases to others within the hospital. At the same time, the normal routine and other special care that a patient who is not in isolation receives should not be less for the patient in isolation. The techniques that follow are considered the minimum to accomplish the primary purpose of isolation and at the same time are designed to help procedures be as simple and practical as possible.

III. Who should be isolated.

Patients with serious infections, potentially serious infections, or suspected serious infections that may be transmitted by airborne routes and/or person-to-person contact should be isolated. Specifically, note the following recommendations.

A. Strict isolation.

    1. *Staphylococcus aureus* pneumonia.

    2. Impetigo.

    3. Heavily draining (frequent penetration of dressings) wound infections caused by any organism.

    4. Major skin infections caused by *S aureus* or group A β-hemolytic streptococci.

    5. Varicella.

      6. Diphtheria.

      7. Plague.

      8. Smallpox or generalized vaccinia.

      9. Congenital rubella.

    10. Patients with pneumonia (or patients with sputum containing a potential pathogen) unable to utilize sanitary cough techniques.

    11. Disseminated *Herpesvirus hominis* (herpes simplex).

    12. Herpes zoster, disseminated. (This disease is probably transmitted primarily by the contact route but may also be transmitted by the airborne route. If there is no possibility of spread to other patients who are immunosuppressed, patients with disseminated herpes zoster may be handled with skin and wound isolation techniques.)

    13. Pulmonary anthrax.

    14. Rabies.

  B. Skin and wound isolation.

      1. All purulent skin and wound infections (except A3 and A4 above).

      2. Ringworm of scalp.

      3. Herpes zoster, localized.

  C. Enteric isolation.

      1. Hepatitis A, B, or unspecified.

      2. *Salmonella*, *Shigella*, *Yersinia*, and *Campylobacter* species.

      3. Cholera.

      4. Typhoid.

      5. Infectious diarrhea and gastroenteritis (viral, bacterial), sporadic and epidemic.

      6. Amebic dysentery.

      7. Poliomyelitis.

  D. Respiratory isolation.

      1. Measles.

      2. Mumps.

      3. Meningococcal infections (including meningitis).

      4. Pertussis.

      5. Rubella.

      6. Tuberculosis, pulmonary.

  E. Protective isolation.—This is optionally available to patients with increased susceptibility to infections. Physicians who admit patients with primary diagnosis of severe burns, leukemia, agranulocytosis, and agammaglobulinemia will be reminded that this service is available if they wish it.

IV. Diagnosis of contagious diseases and policy for disposition to isolation.

  A. The diagnosis of an infectious disease must be made by a physician.

  B. The disposition to isolation must be a physician's order.

C. The attending physician should initiate this procedure whenever a patient becomes infectious.

D. When an infectious condition develops or becomes apparent while a patient is in the hospital, the patient's physician will be notified of this by the head nurse as soon as the condition is discovered. It is expected that the physician will then initiate appropriate directives.

E. Physicians should notify the admitting department of infection states at the time of admission of their patients. The admitting office, in turn, should question the physician concerning the conditions needing isolation on all patients admitted.

F. Patients who do not need isolation at the time of admission but have a high likelihood of requiring isolation within 24 hours should be admitted directly to appropriate rooms (eg, a patient admitted for incision and drainage of an abscess). If the isolation anticipated is skin and wound isolation (eg, for drainage of perirectal abscess), then admission to a ward is permissible.

G. Each patient having, or suspected of having, any of the bacterial diseases above (section III) should have a smear and culture on admission or immediately upon discovery. The nurse epidemiologist or another designated nurse may obtain such cultures (especially from purulent and draining wounds) without a physician's orders. The patient's physician, however, should be notified of this.

H. In the event that an apparent infection state is discovered and the patient's physician cannot be contacted, the chairman of the infection committee (or a representative) should be notified. He or she will then evaluate the situation and issue any necessary directives. If a patient is isolated in this manner, the physician should be notified as soon as he or she can be contacted.

I. In the event a question arises concerning the diagnosis or disposition of patients with contagious diseases, consultation with the chairman of the infection committee (or a designated member) is always available. If a situation arises in which the chairman of the infection committee is of the opinion that a given patient should be isolated and the attending physician declines to do so, the chairman of the committee has the authority to isolate the patient.

V. When disposition out of isolation occurs.

A. Patient is discharged from the hospital.

B. There is clinical improvement accompanied by negative bacterial cultures (bacterial infections).

C. State of infectivity has passed (viral infection).

D. Drainage stops.

E. For any questions concerning disposition, contact the epidemiology department.

ISOLATION PROCEDURES

I. General considerations.

    A. Hand-washing is the single most effective means of preventing not only the occurrence of infection but also the dissemination or spread of infection.

    B. Gowns are worn to provide mechanical protection of personnel engaging in care that necessitates physical contact with the patient and/or unit.

    C. Patient charts are never to be taken into isolation units.

        1. Mark type of isolation above temperature on graphic sheet when isolation is begun.

        2. Mark isolation "dc'ed" when isolation is terminated.

        3. Mark nursing care plan when isolation is begun and terminated.

    D. When returning equipment to central supply for sterilization, do not use wax-coated, red nylon, or any plastic bags. Do use large or small brown paper bags. Items that are too large for brown paper bags may be put into a cloth laundry bag (not red nylon). Tape paper bags closed or tie the laundry bags closed.

    E. Dust, grease, organic material, and other contaminants left on articles interfere with the sterilization process. Therefore, ALL ARTICLES FROM ISOLATION MUST BE THOROUGHLY CLEANED *BEFORE* THEY ARE SENT TO CENTRAL SUPPLY FOR STERILIZATION.

    F. Place red and white ISOLATION label across the front of the chart on all patients in isolation. Write the type of isolation (ie, skin and wound, enteric) on the label.

    G. All patients who are to be isolated should have a full explanation of the purpose and meaning of being in isolation. This should be done so as not to alarm the patient and therefore should be done by the physician or nurse.

    H. When a patient is to be transferred to an isolation room, rooms on the same unit or floor should be used if at all possible. Transfers to different floors for purposes of isolation are discouraged.

    I. Nurse epidemiologist will make rounds on all isolation patients, keep records, and report daily to the hospital epidemiologist. During rounds the NE will observe the adequacy of infection control and isolation techniques.

    J. It is realized that situations will arise in which diagnosis and disposition are not adequately covered by the above guidelines. The infection committee is always available for consultation for such situations.

II. Strict isolation.

    A. Definition.—Strict isolation is the practice of techniques designed to prevent the transmission of the most contagious diseases in which direct contact, fomites, and air are recognized means of communicability.

    B. Location.—Private room with running water necessary.

C. Procedure.
 1. Hand-washing.
  a. Turn faucets on.
  b. Lather hands with soap and water; avoid using bar soap if possible.
  c. Wash hands thoroughly, using friction on all surfaces.
  d. Rinse under running water, holding hands down.
  e. Dry with clean paper towel from dispenser.
  f. Turn off faucets with paper towel to avoid contamination of hands.
 2. Use of gown.
  a. To put on: Put gown on with opening at back and tie strings at neck. Lap gown at back to cover uniform and tie.
  b. To remove: Untie strings at waist.
  c. Wear gown one time only and discard in plastic water-soluble bag in room.
  d. Wash hands after removing gown just prior to leaving the room.
 3. Care of linen.
  a. Avoid vigorous movements when changing linen to prevent scattering of bacteria.
  b. Use cotton blankets.
  c. Have plastic protectors on pillows.
  d. Place soiled linen in clear plastic water-soluble bag inside room, being careful to wrap wet linen inside dry linen *before* placing in bag (eg, wrap washcloth in towel).
  e. Place clear plastic bag with soiled linen into red laundry bag held by person outside the room.
  f. DO NOT TAPE LAUNDRY BAG, take directly to laundry chute.
 4. Care of food and dishes.
  a. Notify dietary department and obtain "Isolation Tray."
  b. Remove all metal containers and lids from tray. DO NOT TAKE INTO ROOM.
  c. Pour coffee, tea, and other hot liquids into styrofoam cups.
  d. Gown before taking tray into room and assisting patient.
  e. Discard liquid waste into sink or toilet.
  f. Discard solid food waste and the disposable food containers, silverware, and tray (which is folded) into plastic bag.
  g. Place plastic bag into paper bag held by a person outside the room. (Coffee pot, if mistakenly taken into room, is to be autoclaved. Place tongue blade in coffee pot to keep lid open before double bagging for central supply.)
 5. Care of drinking water.
  a. Leave disposable plastic water pitcher and disposable cup in room. (If patient prefers a glass instead of a disposable cup, replace with clean glass every morning.) Double bag glass and send to central supply.
  b. Replace liner in pitcher daily before filling with fresh water from sink.

      c. Ice may be obtained by using disposable liner at ice machine. Obtain ice before gowning and entering room.

6. Taking and recording vital signs.
    a. Temperature.
        i. Keep thermometer in container filled with 70% alcohol.
        ii. Containers are to be cleaned in room every two days and refilled with 70% alcohol.
        iii. Rinse thermometer with cold water *before* taking patient's temperature.
        iv. After use, wipe the thermometer with a cotton ball and wash with cold water. Dry and place in container.
    b. Blood pressure.
        i. For repeated blood pressure measurements, requisition central supply for portable blood pressure apparatus and leave it in room until isolation is terminated.
        ii. For admission blood pressure, use floor machine and stethoscope. To remove from room, discard cloth cuff into plastic laundry bag, clean all surfaces of sphygmomanometer and stethoscope with 70% alcohol, and place directly outside room to be taken back to clean area.
    c. Vital signs.
        i. Record all vital signs on scratch paper in room.
        ii. Tape paper to an area easily seen from doorway.
        iii. Transcribe onto clean scratch paper and/or patient's chart after leaving room.

7. Collection of specimens.
    a. Obtain specimen from patient.
    b. Wipe outside of covered specimen container with 70% alcohol while in room.
    c. Place specimen on clean paper towel just inside doorway.
    d. After leaving room, place specimen in paper bag, label contents, mark "Isolation," and send directly to laboratory.

8. Signing documents.
    a. Place clean paper towels on overbed table.
    b. Place documents on paper towels and have patient sign.
    c. Take document directly out of room after disposing of gown and washing hands.

9. Transportation of patients.
    a. With two sheets, cover stretcher or wheelchair outside of room.
    b. Don clean isolation gown and take stretcher or wheelchair into room and assist patient onto conveyance.
    c. Move stretcher or wheelchair away from bed.
    d. Remove isolation gown and wash hands.
    e. Fold sheet that was next to bed up over patient with his or her hands and arms tucked inside, taking care not to touch contaminated side of sheet.
    f. Move patient to hallway and wrap second sheet over patient.

g. All wheelchairs and stretchers must be cleaned with Vesphene after use. DO NOT USE CONVEYANCE FOR ANOTHER PATIENT UNTIL IT HAS BEEN CLEANED.
h. Inform department to which patient is being sent that he or she is in isolation.

10. Visitors.
   a. Report to nursing station before entering room. Should be informed of the purpose of isolation and instructed in proper technique of gowning and hand-washing and the need to avoid direct contact with patient.
   b. Should be kept to two visitors at a time.
   c. Visitors purses.—Place in open paper bag just before entering room; take into room; after removing gown and washing hands, visitor may just reach into paper bag for purse.

11. Care of articles and equipment used in strict isolation.
   a. Patient's clothing.—*Do not take clothing with patient into isolation if patient is being transferred to another room for isolation.* If clothing is present in room when isolation begins, remove clothing and place in paper bag and label, or give clothing to family with instructions to wash separately. Have family bring clean clothing when patient is to be discharged.
   b. Leather articles (shoes, wallet, belt, etc).—Wipe outside of articles with Vesphene upon termination of isolation.
   c. Transfer of patient's articles from one room to another.
      i. Cover cart or wheelchair with two sheets.
      ii. Place articles on cart.
      iii. Wrap inner sheet over articles first and then wrap outer sheet and proceed to transfer articles.
   d. Flowers, letters, cards, magazines, and books.—May be sent home with family if patient so requests. Encourage that these articles be discarded rather than sent home with patient. Use of hard-bound books is to be discouraged.
   e. Clocks, radios, and similar articles.—Wipe with alcohol and transfer with patient or send home with family.
   f. Utensils.—These utensils are transferred with patient.
      i. Bath basin.
      ii. Emesis basin.
      iii. Soap dish.
      iv. Tooth mug.
      v. Drinking water containers (carafes).
      vi. Water glass.
      vii. Bedpan.
      viii. Urinal.

III. Skin and wound isolation.

   A. Definition.—Skin and wound isolation is the practice of techniques designed to prevent the transmission of infections dependent on direct person-to-person contact for their communicability.

B. Location.—Private room desirable; open ward with running water can be used.

C. Equipment.

   1. Isolation card.—Hang outside door only if patient is in private room. Attach to foot of bed if patient is in open ward.

   2. Clear plastic water-soluble bags for linen, from central supply.

   3. Paper bags for double bagging equipment, from supply cart.

   4. Sterile disposable gloves.—Take into room as needed.

   5. If patient is in ward, instruct him or her to use toilet seat covers.

   6. Red laundry bags.

   7. Patient's gown.

D. Procedure.

   1. Patient gown.—To be worn by all persons having direct contact with patient or bed (ie, morning care, changing linen, dressing changes).

   2. Gloves.—To be worn by *all* persons changing the dressing or having direct contact with the infected area.

   3. Wash hands with soap and water before and after direct contact with patient.

   4. Masks are not necessary.

   5. Dressings and dressing tray.—Gloves to be worn always.

   6. Linen.

      a. Avoid vigorous movements when changing linen to prevent scattering of bacteria.

      b. Pillows are to have plastic protectors.

      c. Double-bag technique.

   7. Laboratory, x-ray, and IV.—Inform lab, x-ray, and IV personnel that patient is in skin and wound isolation. Mark requisition "S AND W ISOLATION" when transcribing orders. Personnel to wear patient gown when drawing blood, starting IV, or taking x-rays.

   8. Equipment needed.

      a. Thermometers.

      b. Dishes and drinking water.

      c. Sphygmomanometer and stethoscope.

      d. Needles and syringes.

   9. No special precautions.

      a. Thermometers.

      b. Dishes and drinking water.

      c. Sphygmomanometer and stethoscope.

      d. Needles and syringes.

      e. Urine and feces.

      f. Specimens.

      g. Clothing and personal effects.

  10. Transportation of patients.—Before transporting patient, the infected area should be adequately covered and dressings changed.

  11. Patient's chart.—Mark "IN S AND W ISOLATION" above

temperature or graphic sheet when isolation is begun and "S AND W ISOLATION DC'ED" when isolation is terminated. Also write on nursing care plan.

  12. Visitors.—Same procedures as for strict isolation.

IV. Enteric isolation.

  A. Definition.—Enteric isolation is the practice of techniques designed to prevent the transmission of disease dependent on the fecal-oral route for communicability.

  B. Location.—Private room with bathroom preferred. If absolutely necessary, may use open ward with bathroom.

  C. Equipment.

    1. Isolation card.—Hang on outside of door *only* if patient is in private room. Attach to foot of bed if patient is in open ward.

    2. Disposable gloves.—Keep in room.

    3. Paper bags.—Do not keep in patient's room. Take into room as needed.

    4. Clear plastic water-soluble bags for linen.—Take into room as needed.

    5. Red laundry bags.—Do not keep in patient's room.

    6. Gowns.

    7. Disposable box for needles and syringes.—Keep in room. For use with patients who have serum or infectious hepatitis.

  D. Procedure.

    1. Patient gowns are to be worn by all persons having direct contact with patient or bed and by all persons handling articles contaminated by feces. Lab, x-ray, and IV personnel must wear patient gown when drawing blood, starting IV, or taking x-ray. *Note:* Fresh blood is considered a possible contaminant in patients with serum and infectious hepatitis.

    2. Gloves are worn by all persons having contact with heavily contaminated articles (ie, bedpans, soiled linen).

    3. Wash hands with soap and water immediately before and after direct contact with patient or unit.

    4. Masks are not necessary.

    5. Needles and syringes.—Procedure for patients with serum or infectious hepatitis.

      a. Place disposable container in room for needles and syringes.

      b. Inform lab, x-ray, and IV of all patients with hepatitis. Mark requisition "ENTERIC ISOLATION—HEPATITIS."

    6. Linens.

      a. Avoid all vigorous movements to avoid aerosols of bacteria.

      b. Pillows are to have plastic protectors.

      c. Use double-bag technique.

    7. Specimens.

       a. Urine.—No special precautions.

       b. Stool.—No special precautions but label "ENTERIC ISOLA-TION" before sending to laboratory. (If outside of container is contaminated, double bag and label as such.)

       c. Blood.—No special precautions, but label "ENTERIC ISOLA-TION—HEPATITIS" before sending to laboratory.

  8. Transportation of patients.—Usually no special precautions. If patient is incontinent:

       a. Double sheet vehicle.

       b. Do not use vehicle for any other patient before cleaning with Vesphene.

       c. Double bag linen.

  9. Dishes.—Usually no special precautions, depending on age and reliability of patient.

  10. No special precautions.

       a. Urinal.

       b. Sphygmomanometer and stethoscope.

       c. Dressings.

       d. Thermometers.

       e. Drinking water and glass.

       f. Clothing and personal effects.

  11. Patient's chart.

       a. Mark "IN ENTERIC ISOLATION" above temperature or graphic sheet when isolation is begun and "ENTERIC ISOLA-TION DC'ED" when isolation is terminated.

       b. Also enter on nursing care plan.

  12. Visitors.

       a. Should be limited to two persons.

       b. Should be informed of the purpose of isolation and instructed not to come in contact with patient's linen, toilet articles, and bathroom.

V. Respiratory isolation.

  A. Purpose.—To prevent transmission of organisms by means of droplets and droplet nuclei that are coughed, sneezed, or breathed into the environment.

  B. Location.—Private room required.

  C. Procedure.

    1. Gowns and gloves are not necessary.

    2. Masks are worn when patient is uncooperative, unable, or unwilling to use proper cough technique.

    3. Hands must be washed on entering and leaving the room.

    4. Dressings and tissues.—Double bag and discard.

    5. Visitors are limited to two persons at a time. Nursing personnel should instruct visitors in the wearing of masks, if indicated, and the

necessity for adherence to isolation. The patient should also wear a mask when visitors are in the room, if indicated.

    6. No special precautions.

       a. Needles.

       b. Sphygmomanometer and stethoscope.

       c. Urine and feces.

       d. Thermometers.

       e. Linen and clothing.

       f. Books and personal items.

       g. Dishes.

    7. Transporting patients.—Notify department of patient's disease. Patient should wear a mask.

VI. Respiratory isolation for patients with tuberculosis.

    A. Teach patient scrupulous cough techniques.

       1. Cover patient's mouth with disposable paper tissue when he or she is coughing, raising sputum, or sneezing.

       2. Tissues should be placed in paper bags at bedside. Bags should be placed in plastic-lined wastepaper basket.

    B. Hospital personnel require a mask and gown only when intimate contact with an uncooperative patient is necessary.

    C. No special care for laundry, dishes, books.

    D. Visitors need not be subjected to restrictions or special precautions.

    E. Hand-washing is efficient in removing organisms possibly picked up from fomites or direct contact with infectious sputum or other dischàrges.

VII. Protective (reverse) isolation.

    A. Definition.—This is optionally available to patients with increased susceptibility to infection. Physicians who admit patients with primary diagnosis of severe burns, leukemia, agranulocytosis, or agammaglobulinemia will be reminded that this service is available if they wish it.

    B. Location.—Private room with bathroom necessary. Keep door closed.

    C. Equipment (from central supply).

       1. Isolation card.—Hang on outside of door.

       2. Sterile linen packs.

          a. Gown pack.—Includes sterile cap, gown, and mask. Keep on cart outside room.

          b. Bed pack.—Take pack *into room before opening.*

       3. Sterile gloves.

       4. Shoe covers (optional).

    D. Procedure.

       1. Gowns, sterile.—To be worn by all persons entering room.

       2. Caps, sterile.—To be worn by all persons who have direct contact with patient.

3. Masks, sterile.—To be worn by all persons entering room.

4. Gloves.—To be worn by all personnel who have direct contact with patient.

5. Wash hands with soap and water *before* entering room and on leaving the room.

6. All linen in contact with patient should be sterile prior to use. Keep sterile linen pack *inside* room. No special precautions after use.

7. Clean sphygmomanometer and stethoscope before taking into room and leave in room until isolation discontinued, if possible.

8. Transportation of patients should be kept to a minimum to avoid exposure to any source of infection.

9. Patient's chart.—Mark "IN PROTECTIVE ISOLATION" above temperature on graphic sheet when isolation is begun and "PROTECTIVE ISOLATION DC'ED" when isolation is terminated. Mark nursing care plan.

10. No special precautions.
    a. Needles and syringes.
    b. Dressings and instruments.
    c. Thermometers.
    d. Dishes.
    e. Urine and feces.
    f. Specimens.
    g. Clothing and personal effects.

11. Visitors should be limited to two persons. Visitors should be informed of the purpose of isolation and instructed in use of sterile cap, gown, and mask.

Note: Remember that procedures that are ordinarily innocuous can result in a most serious infection among this group of patients.

VIII. Isolation procedure for emergency department.

    A. Purpose.—To isolate, protect, and minimize risk to emergency department patients and personnel from the transmission of contagious diseases.

    B. Location.—The shower room is the room of choice for isolation of emergency department patients.

    C. Equipment (to be kept outside of room).

      1. Roll stand with basin with disinfectant solution.
      2. Rectal gloves.
      3. Washcloths.
      4. Chair with clean linen bag.
      5. Kick bucket bags.
      6. Sterilizer tray.
      7. Clean set of linen, water-soluble linen bag.
      8. Open sterilizer door in utility room.

D. Procedure.

1. Prior to putting patient in shower room, remove all but necessary equipment, ie, movable cart with supplies, chairs, oxygen tanks, outside of room.

2. Make sure all supplies that will be needed for procedure and also for cleanup are outside of room, ie, refer to Equipment section above.

3. Put patient in room and explain procedure. Obtain necessary vital signs and record them on emergency department chart.

4. Assist patient to comfortable position and place Chux pads underneath affected part, eg, incision and drainage (I & D), debridement.

5. Assist physician with procedure.

6. After procedure, "dirty" personnel should put on rectal gloves and proceed to clean room.

   a. Strip linen from stretcher and place in water-soluble linen hamper in shower room.
   b. Wash stretcher, kick bucket, and all washable objects with disinfectant.
   c. Place dirty instruments in disinfectant solution and then place these instruments in sterilizer tray. This includes sharp objects (needles, knife, blades). After items are sterilized, dispose of items in regular manner.
   d. Empty disinfectant solution in hopper in utility room.
   e. Take sterilizer trays with empty basin and place in sterilizer in utility room. Have "clean" personnel close sterilizer door and turn sterilizer on to flash cycle.
   f. Place water-soluble linen bag inside clean linen bag. Be very careful not to contaminate outside of clean linen bag.
   g. Place full plastic waste container inside clean plastic bag. Take off rectal gloves and toss in bag. Be very careful not to contaminate outside of plastic bag.
   h. Throw double-bagged trash and linen into appropriate receptacles.
   i. Restore shower room to proper order.

IX. Maintenance and engineering isolation procedure.
Check with unit nurse before entering the patient's room. When it becomes necessary to perform maintenance repairs in an isolation room, the following procedures shall be used. The maintenance engineer shall follow the dress code appropriate for the type of isolation (see Isolation Procedure): strict—gown, mask, and gloves; respiratory—mask; protective—sterile gown, mask, and gloves; enteric—gown, gloves if in contact with bathroom facilities, patient, or patient's bed; skin and wound—gown and gloves if in contact with patient or patient's bed.

A. Entering the isolation room.—Follow isolation procedure. Hands must be washed before and after entering the room.

B. Leaving the isolation room.—Follow isolation procedure.

C. After entering strict, respiratory, or protective isolation room, analyze the scope of repair work. Have "clean" person outside room to provide all tools or parts necessary to effect repairs. This is not necessary for skin and wound or enteric isolation. All equipment and tools introduced to the room are considered contaminated. Keep a minimum quantity of tools to do the job.

    D.   Sterilization of equipment.

        1.   After repairs are completed, wipe all tools and parts with phenolic solution. All equipment is considered contaminated.

        2.   For strict and respiratory isolation, place equipment that is *heat sensitive* in double plastic bags to be gas sterilized. If in doubt about heat sensitivity, prepare items for gas sterilization.

        3.   For strict and respiratory isolation, place equipment that can tolerate extreme heat in double bags (*not plastic*) for steam sterilization.

        4.   Double-bagging technique.—For strict and respiratory isolation; not necessary for protective, skin and wound, or enteric isolation.

            a.   After equipment is wiped and placed in appropriate sterilization bag, carry bagged equipment to the door.

            b.   Place in cuffed bag held by "clean" person outside patient's room.

            c.   "Clean" person will fold over top edge of bag and fasten with tape; label bag as to contents, instructions, and location; and send to central supply.

    E.   Equipment that cannot be repaired in the room and is too large to be autoclaved, such as beds, should be wiped with phenolic solution and transported to the repair shop.

    F.   Direct all isolation questions or problems to the nurse in the units or to the epidemiology department.

X. Nursery isolation procedure.

    A.   Purpose.—To isolate and protect nursery from an infant whose mother has herpes or is suspected of having herpes, or from any infant with a staphylococcal infection or unusual skin lesions (draining wounds).

    B.   Equipment.

        1.   Warmer or isolette.

        2.   Isolation room.—To completely isolate infant.

        3.   Personnel to care for infant.—To prevent contamination of regular nursery and its supplies. It is imperative to have a one-to-one nurse–patient relationship.

        4.   Gown.—To protect clothing from contamination.

        5.   IV, standard.—Hang gown with side to baby folded in. Gown to be changed every eight hours.

        6.   Gloves, mask, and cap as indicated. See hospital policy concerning isolation.

    C.   Procedure.

        1.   Set up equipment. Prepare for admission of infant in advance. All supplies should be stocked in the isolation room, including linen, to be used only by the isolated infant.

2. Gown upon infant's arrival to protect clothing from contamination. Remind staff of importance for them to change their contaminated clothing.

3. Use careful hand-washing to protect baby and self against contamination. Hands should be washed prior to handling infant, after handling infant, prior to gown removal, and before leaving isolation room.

4 Obtain culture at physician's discretion to identify organisms present. Take a culture from any draining lesions or pustules for culture, sensitivity, and smear.

5. Notify pediatrician of isolation and its reason. Obtain further orders.

6. Notify hospital nurse epidemiologist so that the case may be followed.

7. Infants in isolation are not to be taken out of the isolation room.

8. Isolation is to be carried out according to the isolation policy of the hospital.

D. Clinical record.

1. Chart on nursing record the date and time isolation was started. Also mark on Kardex.

2. Chart on progress record. Chart in *red* as this is a problem.

XI. Nursery: Segregation procedure.

A. Purpose.—To prevent cross-contamination of infants already admitted to nursery from these sources.

1. Infants born outside the unit.

2. Infants readmitted or admitted from other hospitals.

3. Infants whose mothers have diarrhea and/or nausea and vomiting.

4. Mothers of infants with temperature of 101 F orally at any time.

5. Ruptured membranes for longer than 24 hours.

6. Infants of mothers who have been ill within 24 hours of delivery.

B. Equipment

1. Warmer.—To isolate infant.

2. Clean gown.—To protect clothing from contamination. Gown should be changed every shift.

3. IV, standard.—Hang gown with dirty side inward to prevent cross-contamination.

C. Essential steps in procedure.

1. Set up equipment. Prepare for admission of infant to prevent cross-contamination upon infant's arrival. Equipment should be placed four to five feet from other units. All supplies needed for infant care, including linen, should be stocked in the warmer.

2. Gown upon infant's arrival to protect clothing from contamination. Remind staff of their possible contamination.

3. Careful hand-washing is imperative to control cross-contamination. Hands should be cleaned prior to handling infants, after handling, prior to gown removal, and after gown is removed.

4. Obtain cultures at physician's discretion to identify organisms that may be present. Check physician's standing orders prior to admission to determine whether cultures are needed. Routinely take cultures from infants with ruptured membranes for longer than 24 hours and from those born outside of the unit. May culture aspirate, ear, and/or cord and send for culture and sensitivity and smear. See also the procedure dealing with readmission.

5. Notify pediatrician to inform of the infant's segregation and its reason and for possible further orders.

6. Infants are to remain segregated and be kept in nursery until pediatrician removes segregation. A physician must order when the infant is to go out to mother.

7. Notify assistant director of nursing service.

8. Notify hospital nurse epidemiologist. If the infant has a communicable disease, then the employee health nurse will need to be notified also.

D. Clinical record.

1. Chart on nursing record the date and time isolation was started. Also mark on Kardex.

2. Chart on progress record. Chart in *red* as this is a problem.

XII. Admitting infants with prolonged rupture of membranes for longer than 24 hours.

A. Purpose.—To initiate protective segregation for the high-risk infant with prolonged rupture of membranes for longer than 24 hours.

B. Equipment.

1. Armstrong warmer.—If in distress, admit infant to radiant warmer.

2. IV pole with gown.

3. Admitting equipment.

4. Sterile culture tube.

5. Sterile DeLee trap.—For gastric aspirate.

6. Appropriate laboratory requisitions.

7. Crib sheet placed at desk area. Nothing that comes in contact with the infant or the infant's bed should leave that area without being washed with Vesphene.

C. Procedure.

1. Admit to Armstrong warmer unless in distress. Notification should be received from staff of pending admittance of infant with prolonged rupture of membranes. Armstrong warmer will be the infant's unit until segregation is discontinued by the physician.

2. Notify physician of segregation and culture done as per physician's preference. *An infant must remain in the nursery* while in segregation unless physician orders that the infant may go out to the mother. The infant's unit must be four to five feet from any other unit.

3. Clean gown on IV pole near infant's warmer is to be worn by all personnel who come in contact with the infant or unit. The gown is to be changed every shift. Gown is to be hung contaminated side in. Wash hands prior to and after gown is put on and removed.

4. Obtain cultures.

    a. Gastric aspirate.—Culture and sensitivity, gram stain stat. Check individual physician's orders. Use a DeLee trap that is sterile and will contain specimen. If DeLee is done in the delivery room, the nurse should bring the specimen into the nursery with the infant.

    b. Ear swab culture.—Culture and gram stain stat. Carry to the laboratory immediately. Gram stain results should be called to the nursery by the laboratory. Report to physician the results of stain.

5. Check and record infant's temperature and environment temperature. A sudden change in temperature (usually hypothermia) is a vital clinical sign of sepsis. The nurse should be familiar with all signs and symptoms of sepsis.

D. Chart on the clinical record flow sheet. Keep crib sheet at desk area as the infant's warmer is in segregation. Record when segregation is started and discontinued on nurse's graph.

Immediate control measures are not limited to isolation procedures. For example, the discovery of a nosocomial epidemic demands quick action to bring the outbreak under control. Unlike isolation policies, there are no existing policies that reflexly set into action measures to control an epidemic. Outbreaks vary considerably in their epidemiology. Policies should exist that authorize appropriate, thorough, and rapid investigation of outbreaks as well as subsequent implementation of appropriate measures to end them.

PROCEDURAL CONTROL MEASURES

Procedural control involves policies and procedures developed and implemented by the ICC in response to surveillance information accumulated over a period of time. On the basis of data provided by the surveillance of practices and infections and analysis of interrelationships among them, it is often possible to discover deficiencies in practice that are allowing a higher than necessary infection rate. Once such areas are uncovered, the development of appropriate corrective procedures and their implementation should be natural consequences.

EMPLOYEE HEALTH SERVICE

Not only are hospital personnel susceptible to infections occurring in patients, but once infected, they may serve as a source or reservoir to infect patients or other personnel. Maximum cooperation between the employee health service (EHS) and the NE is necessary to minimize the infection risks to and from personnel. Surveillance of infections among employees should be included in the general infection surveillance by the NE. Policies and procedures should be developed and implemented for the disposition of employees with infections. Depending on the nature of such infections, the employee may be allowed to work with no modification of activities, allowed to work with limited or altered activities, or required to abstain from work altogether until the period of infectivity has elapsed.

Most states require at least annual checks of personnel in health care facilities for tuberculosis—by either skin testing or chest x-ray examination. The cost-effectiveness of this probably will vary with the geographic location as well as with the type of population served by the institution.

Prevention of personnel infections should be considered a joint charge of both the EHS and the ICC. In addition to the appropriate disposition of infected patients and personnel, immunization should be advocated when indicated. Across-the-board recommendations in this regard are not rational. Recommendations should be dependent on the endemic and epidemic infection problems in the community. The infection control committee should be cognizant of these and be responsible for making appropriate recommendations. The following, as an example, is the infection control policy for the EHS at St. Vincent Hospital and Medical Center.

INFECTION CONTROL POLICIES FOR EMPLOYEE HEALTH SERVICE

Since an effective infection control program in the hospital requires protection of both patients and personnel, it is essential that the employee health service (EHS) and the hospital epidemiology department cooperate in a program of detection, evaluation, and prevention of infection in hospital personnel. Listed below are some basic policies of infection control for the EHS. Questions or problems not covered by these policies should be directed to the chairman of the infection committee or house epidemiologist.

  I. Pre-employment examinations.

     A. Prospective employees must provide certification from their personal physician giving details of their present health status as well as relevant past history, family history, and infectious disease history.

     B. Prospective employees who have no personal physician may visit primary care center physicians to obtain such a certificate.

C. Routine chest x-ray.

D. Intermediate strength purified protein derivative (PPD) test (unless prospective employee is a known positive reactor).

E. Routine laboratory work (complete blood cell count).

F. Serum HBsAg on all with history of hepatitis.

G. Rubella antibody test on women of child-bearing age.

II. Annual examination.

A. Repeat PPD skin test on all employees whose previous test results were negative or less than 1.0 cm in diameter.

B. Chest x-ray for all employees who are positive PPD reactors (old or current converters).

C. All PPD converters or employees with abnormal chest x-ray findings must consult their personal physician. Those without personal physicians may consult primary care center physicians.

III. Infections reportable to EHS.

All employees should report infections to EHS or their department head. Each department head should report such infections to EHS and be attuned to possible infections that have not yet been reported. EHS or HE should be contacted in these situations.

A. Employees working in critical care areas (ICU, cardiac recovery room, operating room, nursery) must report all infectious diseases and refrain from working in these areas until the period of infectivity is over (must be cleared through EHS).

B. Cutaneous infections.—Employees with skin infections must report these to EHS, and if their work involves direct or indirect patient contact, they should refrain from this until infection has healed. Personnel with herpetic lesions (cold sores) should refrain from working in the newborn nursery or with immunosuppressed patients on other units.

C. Respiratory infections.—Except for minor colds, respiratory infections should be reported to EHS.

1. Pharyngitis.—Employee should see a physician, get a culture if necessary, and refrain from working (if it involves direct patient contact) until illness is over or after 24 hours of appropriate therapy.

2. Viral infections.—Minor colds and upper respiratory infections unassociated with fever need not be reported routinely and should not be a reason for time off work. Employees who are febrile should be reported to EHS for disposition.

D. Urinary tract infections.—These need not be reported under ordinary circumstances, but employee should see personal physician for appropriate therapy.

E. Gastrointestinal infections.

1. Diarrhea.—Any employee with diarrhea should report to EHS for culture and disposition. Any employee who has patient contact or

works in the food service must refrain from work until the infection has been treated or until the diarrhea has been demonstrated to have a noninfectious cause.

2. Hepatitis.—Any employee who develops hepatitis or jaundice may not work in the hospital. Such persons should report to EHS and to their personal physician for disposition. A blood test for HBsAg should be performed. Employees may return to work when well (certified by physician). Chronic HBsAg carriers or employees who have recovered from hepatitis B but remain persistently HBsAg positive should refrain from working in sensitive areas, namely, heart-lung bypass areas, dialysis units, and food preparation areas.

IV. Contact with contagious infectious diseases.

A. Tuberculosis.—This disease is not highly contagious but usually requires fairly long-term or intimate contact with infected persons. This type of contact can occur in the hospital in cases where the infection is not diagnosed until some days after admission and the usual prophylactic measures have not been taken prior to then. In such or similar situations, the following should be done.

1. Close contacts who are PPD-negative.
   a. Those whose last PPD test was more than three months ago should have stat PPD test done.
   b. All should have another PPD test done in six to eight weeks.
   c. If PPD test results remain negative, nothing more need be done.
   d. If PPD results have become positive, such contacts should have a chest x-ray and report to their personal physician for further disposition.

2. Close contacts who are PPD-positive.
   a. Those who are currently taking antibuterculous drugs need do no more.
   b. Those not taking such drugs and whose last chest x-ray was more than three months ago should have an x-ray immediately.
   c. Repeat chest x-ray in eight weeks (not necessary for a above).
   d. Those whose x-rays change or who have suspicious lesions should consult their personal physicians.

B. Hepatitis.—Usually transmitted by fecal-oral route or parenterally.

1. Normal hand-washing is generally considered good prophylaxis against fecal-oral transmission.

2. Prolonged close contact during the early stages of the disease before it is recognized (eg, in family members) may increase the likelihood of such transmission. If the hepatitis is HBsAg-negative, prophylactic gammaglobulin should be administered to such contacts.

3. Parenteral transmission from patients to employees is usually the result of accidents, eg, nicking the skin with a needle after it has been used in a hepatitis patient or oral contamination with such a patient's blood. If the patient's hepatitis is HBsAg-negative, employees suffering such accidental exposure should receive prophylatic gammaglobulin. If it is HBsAg-positive, hepatitis B immune globulin should be considered.

   C. Viral childhood infections.—Most adults have had these infections and are therefore immune; hence, such contacts are inconsequential. If an employee is not certain of having had such previous infections or immunization and is exposed to such an infection (eg, rubella), immediate serologic studies should be performed to establish the immune status of the employee. If the serologic test results are positive, no more need be done. If negative, consideration should be given to gammaglobulin prophylaxis, and careful observations for the first signs of infection are in order.

V. Immunizations.
Mandatory vaccinations are not required at this time. However, certain immunizations are recommended and available through EHS.

   A. Influenza.—Because of the changing antigenic nature of these viruses, employees should be vaccinated annually in the fall against the current epidemic strains.

   B. Diphtheria tetanus.—Recommended every ten years.

   C. Poliomyelitis.—Recommended for all, but particularly for personnel working in pediatrics wards.

   D. Rubella.—Nonimmune women in the child-bearing age who are not pregnant (and who are unlikely to become pregnant within two months) should be vaccinated.

INVOLVEMENT OF OUTSIDE AGENCIES

Hospital epidemiology programs must not operate in isolation from the rest of the community. Free and appropriate communication between the NE of each health care facility and the regional public health authorities is both essential and mutually beneficial. Through such communication, hospital authorities are alerted to infection problems in the community that may affect patients who will require special infection control measures. On the other hand, appropriate early reporting of communicable disease discovered in patients in the hospital can provide public health authorities with critical clues to the discovery of or solution to a community health problem. In addition, public health experts from local or state health departments or the CDC often are willing to help individual hospital officials solve difficult epidemiologic problems. The policies cited here from St. Vincent should be considered the minimum to satisfy current state regulations.

POLICY FOR REPORTING COMMUNICABLE DISEASES

1. Objective.—To assure the prompt and accurate reporting of all communicable diseases, both to those within the hospital who must know for professional reasons and to those external health agencies to whom the hospital is required by law to report.

2. Policy.—All communicable diseases that are diagnosed at St. Vincent Hospital and Medical Center will be reported to the hospital's nurse epidemiologist. The nurse epidemiologist, or in her or his absence, the person designated to replace her or him, shall be responsible for reporting the communicable diseases.

  a. Internal reporting of communicable disease.—The nurse epidemiologist is responsible for informing the hospital epidemiologist, assistant administrator of professional services, chairman of the infection committee, and appropriate department heads of any *extraordinary outbreaks* of communicable disease.

  b. External reporting of communicable disease.—All external reporting of diseases diagnosed at St. Vincent Hospital and Medical Center will conform to the reporting requirements and procedures outlined by the Oregon State Health Division and the Washington County Health Department (procedure follows).

PROCEDURE FOR REPORTING COMMUNICABLE DISEASES

1. The following cases are reportable immediately *by telephone* to the Washington County Health Officer or his or her designee:

Cholera	Relapsing fever
Diarrhea of newborn	(louseborne)
(institutions)	Smallpox
Diphtheria	Syphilis, infectious
Food poisoning	Typhus fever
(including botulism)	(epidemic, louseborne)
Measles	Yellow fever
Plague	

Upon receiving information that any of the above communicable diseases have been diagnosed at St. Vincent Hospital and Medical Center, the nurse epidemiologist will first notify the hospital epidemiologist or designee at St. Vincent Hospital and Medical Center. The nurse epidemiologist will then *telephone* the county. Upon telephoning the reports to Washington County Health Department, the nurse epidemiologist will send in an individual case card to the Washington County Health Department.

2. Any extraordinary outbreaks of communicable disease.—"Extraordinary outbreak of communicable disease" implies an increase in the number of cases of a communicable disease among patients and/or employees in a specific time period. The report of outbreaks need not await final diagnosis but should be made upon suspicion of a problem when an illness manifesting similar symptoms occurs in groups of patients or employees previously not having them. Upon receiving information of any extraordinary outbreaks of communicable disease at St. Vincent Hospital and Medical Center, the nurse epidemiologist will notify the hospital epidemiologist, assistant administrator of professional services, chairman of the infection committee, and appropriate department heads. The nurse epidemiologist will then immediately *telephone* the Washington County Health Department. Upon telephoning the report to

the county health department, the nurse epidemiologist will send in an individual case card to the Washington County Health Department.

3. The following cases are reportable *by individual case card* furnished by the Washington County Health Department:

Amebiasis
Anthrax
Brucellosis
Chancroid
Chickenpox
  (age 16 or over)
Diarrhea, epidemic
Encephalitis
  (infectious and
  postinfectious)
Gonorrhea
Granuloma inguinale
Hepatitis
  (infectious and serum)
Keratoconjunctivitis
  (infectious)
Leprosy
Leptospirosis
Lymphogranuloma venereum
Malaria
Meningitis, aseptic
Meningitis, meningococcal

Ophthalmia neonatorum
Paratyphoid fever
Poliomyelitis
Psittacosis
Q fever
Rabies
  (human and animal cases,
  including animal bites)
Rheumatic fever
Ringworm of scalp
Rocky Mountain spotted fever
Rubella*
Salmonellosis
Scabies
  (schools and institutions)
Shigellosis
Streptococcal infections
Tetanus
Trachoma
Tuberculosis
Tularemia
Typhoid fever

*Cases occurring during the first trimester of pregnancy, congenital anomalies related to rubella, rubella of the newborn.

4. The following are cases reportable only by total number of cases, using the flap of return envelope:

Infectious mononucleosis
Influenza
Mumps
Pertussis
Rubella

INFECTION CONTROL POLICY AND PROCEDURES MANUAL

As mentioned, there should be a manual that contains all the infection control policies and procedures for the hospital—both for the institution in general and for each department or service. These policies should be reviewed periodically (at least annually) and updated as necessary by the ICC. In our institution the infection control manual consists of two massive tomes (two 3-inch, 3-hole, loose-leaf binders). The manual outlines in considerable detail all hospital policies and procedures related to infection control. The table of contents of our manual is given here to provide an insight into the scope of such a guide. Items marked with an asterisk (*) are sections that have been reproduced earlier in this chapter.

ST. VINCENT HOSPITAL AND MEDICAL CENTER INFECTION CONTROL MANUAL
TABLE OF CONTENTS

        c. Infection Control Policies
        d. Isolation Procedures
        e. Standards for Food Service Sanitation
15. Specific Policies and Procedures
        a. Hand-Washing
        b. Dressing Changes
        c. Wound Culture Technique for Obtaining Specimens
        d. Sputum Culture Technique for Obtaining Specimens
        e. Nasotracheal Suctioning
        f. Tracheal, Endotracheal, or Tracheostomy Suctioning
        g. Tracheostomy Incision Care
        h. Urinary Catheterization Procedures
        i. Urinary Retention Catheter Care
        j. Urinary Catheter Irrigation Procedures
        k. Removal of Indwelling Urinary Catheters
        l. Urine Culture Specimens—Method for Procurement
        m. Intravenous Therapy Procedures

            1) Venous Puncture
            2) IV Medications for Syringe
            3) Indwelling Lines
            4) Blood and Blood Products
            5) Hyperalimentation Therapy

        n. Temperature, Pulse, and Respiration Procedure
        o. Decubitus Ulcer Care
        p. Stool Specimens—Method of Procurement
        q. Disposal of Syringes, Sharps, and Needles
        r. Flowers in Hospital Policy
        s. Dress Code and Hand Care Policy—Nursery
        t. Gift Shop Services
        u. Postmortem Procedures

Chapter 9:
Nosocomial Microbes

The agents that cause nosocomial infections are, for the most part, the same as those that produce community-acquired infections. The major difference is one of relative frequency in the two settings. For example, *Streptococcus pneumoniae* is the leading cause of community-acquired bacterial pneumonia but is a less common cause of nosocomial pneumonia, ranking about sixth or seventh in most series. Likewise, the patterns of infections produced by the same species of microbe may differ from the hospital setting to the community. For example, pharyngitis is the most frequent manifestation of *Streptococcus pyogenes* infection in the community, whereas nosocomial *S pyogenes* infections are most often skin and wound infections.

In this chapter, the individual agents that cause nosocomial infections are listed and discussed from an epidemiologic viewpoint with emphasis on the source and mechanisms of infection as well as the patterns and frequency of the infections they cause.

Acinetobacter calcoaceticus: A calcoaceticus var anitratus (synonym: Acinetobacter anitratus, Herellea vaginicola)

This aerobic, oxidase-negative, gram-negative bacillus is a nonfermenting glucose oxidizer. It is ubiquitous in the hospital environment and is isolated most frequently from moist areas such as sinks and humidifiers. Both hospital personnel and inpatients are common carriers of the organism, which is found primarily in the flora of the skin, upper respiratory tract, and genitourinary tract.[86, 523] The incidence of carriers in persons outside the hospital is significantly less—about 8%.[523] Although this organism is of relatively low virulence, bona fide serious infections caused by it are seen with increasing frequency. Examples are pneumonia, intravenous catheter infections, postoperative wound infections, and septicemia.[86, 245, 543, 571] Both human carriers and environmental sources have been documented as major reservoirs. Nosocomial outbreaks, for example, have been traced to an inhalation therapist who was a hand carrier[86] and to room humidifiers.[571] Its low virulence and the prevalence of *A calcoaceticus* in the hospital environment and in the flora of hospitalized patients render interpretation of its isolation from clinical material very difficult at times.

111

Careful correlation and analysis of both clinical and microbiologic informa-tion are required to incriminate this microbe as the cause of an infection. On the other hand, because it can produce infection and is usually resistant to such commonly used antimicrobics as ampicillin, the cephalosporins, and chloramphenicol, its isolation should not be automatically ignored.

Acinetobacter calcoaceticus: A calcoaceticus var lwoffi (synonym: Acinetobacter lwoffi, Mima polymorpha)

This is a related organism but is a nonoxidizer. It is somewhat less prevalent than var anitratus and apparently even less virulent. Nevertheless, true nosocomial infections due to this species have been reported, eg, neonatal meningitis.[6]

Aeromonas hydrophila

This is an oxidase-positive, gram-negative, fermenting facultative bacillus. It is primarily a so-called water organism and occasionally is found in moist areas in the hospital such as sinks and drains.[532] It is not a common component of normal human flora, although it has been found rarely in normal human feces.[348, 630] It has also been implicated occasionally as the cause of gastroenteritis.[348, 630] Clear cases of A hydrophila nosocomial in-fections have included sepsis,[3, 84, 229, 371, 613] meningitis,[489] postoperative wound infections,[637] and urinary tract infections.[140, 637] Many of these have involved compromised hosts.[3, 84, 229, 371, 465] Outbreaks due to A hydrophila in the hospital appear to be rare. Because of the infrequent occurrence of this organism in normal flora, its isolation from clinical material in signifi-cant numbers must be considered seriously.

Alcaligenes faecalis

This aerobic, oxidase-positive, nonfermenting, nonoxidizing, gram-negative motile bacillus with peritrichous flagella is a water organism and may be found occasionally in hospital sinks and drains. It may also be found occasionally as part of human fecal flora. It is of very low virulence but may be a rare cause of nosocomial infections such as neonatal men-ingitis.[553] In ten years of surveillance we have encountered only one case of nosocomial A faecalis infection—sepsis in a patient with colitis of undeter-mined etiology. Its isolation from sources other than blood, cerebrospinal fluid, or urine must be interpreted cautiously. Other species of this genus (A odorans and A denitrificans) presumably exhibit the same low patho-genicity.

Aspergillus species

Aspergillus, a fungus with septate hyphae and characteristic vesicles, sterigmata, and conidia, belongs to the class Ascomycetes. Numerous species are recognized, but those most commonly encountered in clinical material include *A fumigatus*, *A flavus*, *A glaucus*, and *A niger*. These organisms are ubiquitous in the environment both within and outside the hospital. They are readily isolated from the air and horizontal surfaces.[213] They are of quite low pathogenicity, and their infections occur almost exclusively in compromised patients, such as those with malignancies,[399, 671] prosthetic heart valves,[156, 349] cardiac transplants,[255, 533] sarcoidosis,[666] and severe burns,[429] as well as those who are receiving extensive antimicrobial therapy for bacterial infections.[308, 399] Many of the *Aspergillus* infections are pulmonary, particularly those in patients who are immunosuppressed. There is evidence that the contamination of implanted materials is the source of prosthetic valve *Aspergillus* endocarditis.[308] Although *Aspergillus* species infections are treatable by appropriate therapy, they are often fatal because the diagnosis is made too late in the course of the disease—often postmortem. Timely diagnosis of *Aspergillus* species infection is difficult because in patients early in the course of the disease, positive cultures of sputum or blood are uncommon. Also, because of its ubiquity in nature, *Aspergillus* species are common laboratory contaminants. The clinical setting plays an important role here, and treatment often may need to be started without a positive diagnosis if it is to be successful. There is no evidence that *Aspergillus* species infections are communicated from person to person.

Astrovirus

This recently identified viral agent has been incriminated as a cause of diarrhea. An outbreak of nosocomial gastroenteritis in a children's ward was attributed to this agent.[340] The frequency and significance of astrovirus in causing nosocomial infections are not known. Methods for the diagnosis of astrovirus infections are not currently available to clinical microbiology laboratories. Diarrheal outbreaks in health care facilities from which no bacterial agent can be isolated are often of viral origin, and help should be sought from outside agencies such as state health departments or the CDC.

Bacillus species

These species are gram-positive, spore-forming, aerobic or facultative bacilli. Spores of the genus *Bacillus* are ubiquitous in the environment. They are more highly resistant to the killing effect of disinfectant and sterilizing agents than are vegetative microbes, and they may survive for years. Aside from anthrax (which is due to *B anthracis* and does not produce nosocomial infections) and food poisoning (which is due to *B cereus* and is occasionally a nosocomial disease), infections due to *Bacillus* species have been considered rare or questionable. Nevertheless, although their virulence is low, true nosocomial *Bacillus* infections have been documented and have included sepsis,[138, 181, 291, 354] CNS infection,[181, 291, 354] pneumonia,[470] and burn and postoperative wound infections.[463] These are most often due to, but not limited to, *B cereus* and *B subtilis*. Because of the prevalence of these microbes in the environment, their transient presence in human flora, and their frequent occurrence as contaminants, isolation of *Bacillus* species from clinical material must be interpreted with caution. Frequently they are isolated from pus together with other potential pathogens, and their pathogenic role, if any, may be impossible to substantiate. Their isolation from such materials as intravenous catheter tips is rarely significant but must be assessed in light of the clinical situation.[209] Although contagion is not a characteristic of *Bacillus* infection (and hence isolation is not required), rare outbreaks have occurred; eg, an outbreak of *B cereus* bacteremia was traced to a contaminated hemodialysis machine following a change in sterilization procedures.[138]

Bacteroides species

These gram-negative anaerobic bacilli constitute the bulk of the colonic flora in humans and are encountered commonly in the mouth, upper respiratory tract, and genitourinary tract flora. Numerous species are represented in the colonic flora. Since the great majority (if not all) of *Bacteroides* infections are derived from the patient's own flora, they are of endogenous origin.

Bacteroides fragilis

This species is present in relatively small numbers compared with other species, yet it is by far the most common species of *Bacteroides* isolated from infected material. This appears to be due in part to the fact that *B fragilis* is the only species that is encapsulated,[318] and its capsular polysaccharide seems to promote the formation of abscesses.[448] Although *Bacteroides* species are often isolated from clinical material mixed with other aerobic and anaerobic microbes, their pathogenic role in such infections is generally acknowledged. *Bacteroides fragilis* is the most common anaerobic agent causing nosocomial sepsis. These commonly occur in patients with gastrointestinal surgery,[124, 188, 223, 306] genitourinary tract surgery,[124, 223] neoplasms (particularly of abdominal and pelvic organs),[71, 187, 188, 306, 566] diabetes mellitus,[71, 188] decubitus ulcers,[124, 223] and previous steroid, immunosuppressant, and/or antimicrobic therapy.[71, 188] Although nosocomial *Bacteroides fragilis* infections have been documented in all parts of the body, including the central nervous system,[187] they are associated most commonly with abdominal and pelvic events. An interesting epidemiologic study showed an increased colonization of the female genital tract by *Bacteroides* species during the first half of the menstrual cycle, and a significantly higher rate of postoperative infection by *Bacteroides* species in women who had abdominal-pelvic surgery during the first half of their cycle.[431] This suggests that, when possible, elective gynecologic surgery should be relegated to the second half of the menstrual cycle.

In addition to its great importance as a cause of infection, *B fragilis* has increased significance because of its resistance to antimicrobics. Whereas most *Bacteroides* species are susceptible to most antimicrobics, *B fragilis* is susceptible only to chloramphenicol, clindamycin, metronidazole, and high doses of carbenicillin or ticarcillin.

Since *Bacteroides* species infections are of endogenous origin and there is no evidence of cross-infection, there is no need to isolate patients with such infections.

Bacille Calmette Guérin (BCG)

This attenuated strain of *Mycobacterium bovis* is used for vaccination against tuberculosis. BCG has a stimulating effect on the immune response to heterologous antigens. In recent years BCG has been used with some success in the treatment of neoplasms (which have distinct antigens) by either routine vaccination or intralesional injection. One of the complications of this form of cancer immunotherapy has been occasional persistent BCG infections in immunocompromised patients. The infections that are most often seen include local infection,[43, 242] granulomatous hepatitis,[286, 523, 545] and disseminated infections.[226, 459, 508, 521, 523] Although these are clearly iatrogenic nosocomial infections, they are inherent risks accompanying this form of treatment. There is no evidence to indicate that there is person-to-person spread of such infection.

Branhamella catarrhalis

Also called *Neisseria catarrhalis*, this organism is a gram-negative, oxidase-positive diplococcus. It is a normal inhabitant of the oropharynx, and its pathogenic potential is questionable. It may be recovered mixed with other microbes in pus. Cases of prosthetic valve endocarditis have been reported.[482]

Candida species

These yeast-like fungi form pseudohyphae and are speciated on the basis of sporulation and carbohydrate utilization patterns. Members of the genus are widespread in nature and are a common component of normal human microbial flora, although usually in relatively small numbers. Antibiotic therapy readily alters this microbial ecology by suppressing much of the bacterial flora and allowing increased prevalence of yeasts such as *Candida*, thus providing more opportunities for infection by *Candida* species. In addition to antibiotic therapy,[44, 165, 453, 456, 644] other underlying factors predisposing to *Candida* infections include immunosuppression, [144, 165, 173, 421, 453, 564] intravenous implements—especially total parenteral nutrition,[24, 165, 197, 453, 513, 517, 644] underlying malignancies,[165, 173, 386, 421] and diabetes mellitus.[165] Oral colonization by *Candida* species is also significantly increased in persons with diabetes and correlates directly with the blood glucose level at the time the culture sample is taken.[442] Although almost any type of infection can be caused by *Candida* species, there is often a pattern of particular underlying factors and types of nosocomial *Candida* infections. Gastrointestinal and pulmonary candidiasis are common complications in patients whose malignancies are being treated with antibiotics and chemotherapeutic agents.[173, 386, 456] Infective endocarditis due to *Candida* species is commonly associated with patients who have prosthetic heart valves and narcotic abuse.[324, 395, 642] Candidemia and sepsis are often secondary to intravenous therapy, particularly hyperalimentation,[24, 165, 644] and this often can be suspected or diagnosed clinically by observing the characteristic endophthalmitis commonly associated with candidemia. [165, 197, 644] Removal of the intravenous line is the primary therapeutic step and may be all that is required. Contamination of equipment used in the preparation of IV solutions or additives may lead to outbreaks of candidemia.[480] *Candida* peritonitis is frequently associated with peritoneal dialysis.[44, 287] Other forms of nosocomial *Candida* infections include meningitis,[47, 144] osteomyelitis,[564] and deep-seated infections involving the kidney,[456] brain,[456, 513] and heart.[456]

Paralleling the prevalence in the normal flora, candidal infections are most often caused by *C albicans*, which accounts for about 75% of such infections. *C tropicalis* and *C parapsilosis* are seen with intermediate frequency as causes of infection, and only rarely are other species such as *C guilliermondi*, *C krusei*, and *C pseudotropicalis* found in such circumstances.

Because of the prevalence of *Candida* species in the human flora, particularly in persons who are receiving antimicrobial drugs, the differentiation between colonization and infection is often extremely difficult—especially since, because of the debilitated state of many infected patients, the usual clinical signs and symptoms of infection are absent. As a result, many infections are not diagnosed antemortem. On the other hand, the routine indiscriminate treatment of "possible" *Candida* infections cannot be encouraged because of the serious potential side effects of the drugs currently in use—amphotericin B with its serious nephrotoxic potential, and flucytosine to which *Candida* species rapidly develop resistance. There is increasing evidence that serologic tests may be helpful in this differentiation between colonization and infection.[234, 281, 441, 599] To date the major problems are conflicting reports, lack of standardization, and the unavailability of practical tests for routine clinical use.

Except in uncommon instances,[480] nosocomial *Candida* species infections are of endogenous origin with no recognized cross-infection potential.

Chlamydia trachomatis

This tiny (0.3μ) bacterium-like microorganism requires an intracellular environment for growth. It is the cause of inclusion conjunctivitis and the most common cause of nongonococcal urethritis. It is a common inhabitant of the female genital tract—either as a colonizer or as an infecting agent. Until recently, *C trachomatis* had not been considered a cause of nosocomial infection. However, it has now been incriminated as a cause of neonatal conjunctivitis and pneumonitis.[53, 210, 244, 266] These infections are presumably acquired during passage of the infant through an infected or colonized birth canal. The exact prevalence and significance of this nosocomial problem are uncertain. The major difficulty for most institutions has been the unavailability of simple, practical means of diagnosis. Characteristic intracytoplasmic inclusions in conjunctival scrapings are diagnostic when found, but for the diagnosis of chlamydial pneumonitis, more sophisticated methods are required. Outbreaks are not recognized, and transmission from infant to infant within the nursery has not been described.

Citrobacter species

This genus of gram-negative facultative bacteria belongs to the family *Enterobacteriaceae*. Members of this genus, primarily *C freundii* and *C diversus*, are normal inhabitants of the intestinal tract but usually in small numbers. They are often isolated from clinical specimens, usually mixed with other species, and their pathogenic role in the infectious process is often questionable. Nevertheless, documented nosocomial infections due to *Citrobacter* species do occur and include urinary tract infections,[18, 279, 304] wound infections,[18, 241, 304] and septicemia.[18, 241] Of particular concern has been the occasional report of *C diversus* meningitis outbreaks in premature and special-care baby units.[251, 257, 504] The epidemiology of these outbreaks has been studied but remains poorly understood. In one outbreak in which there were three cases during a six-month period, 64 infants were colonized with *C diversus* (umbilicus and/or stool) but were not infected. No carriers were found among the staff, and all environmental cultures were negative.[504] Although not documented, it must be assumed that the infant-to-infant spread occurred via staff hands. Whereas skin and wound isolation is normally sufficient for patients with *Citrobacter* infections, in outbreaks, strict isolation should be considered, particularly in nurseries.

Clostridium difficile

The normal ecology of this anaerobic gram-positive, spore-forming bacillus is not yet well understood. It has been demonstrated to be part of the fecal flora of normal neonates[347] and is probably present in very low numbers in many adults. It has been isolated from patients who have antimicrobic-associated pseudomembranous colitis.[40, 224, 347] A toxin recovered from the feces of such patients is apparently identical with the toxin produced by *C difficule* and is characterized by producing cytotoxicity in human amnion cell cultures[40, 224] and producing fatal enterocolitis in hamsters[40, 347]; it is neutralized by antitoxin to *C sordellii*.[40, 224, 346, 507] *C difficile* is often resistant to clindamycin, the drug most often associated with pseudomembranous colitis. It is suggested that the disease is due to increased toxin production by a relative overgrowth of *C difficile* resulting from selective inhibition of other major constituents of the normal fecal flora by antibiotics such as clindamycin. Although the disease is often nosocomial, it may not be an infection in the true sense of the word.

Clostridium perfringens

A gram-positive, anaerobic, spore-forming bacillus, this organism, whose resistant spores are ubiquitous in nature, is normally found in the vegetative form in the intestinal tracts of humans and animals. Although gas gangrene following major traumatic injuries is the most dramatic and widely recognized form of *C perfringens* infection, nosocomial infections also occur occasionally and may be equally dramatic. The gastrointestinal tract appears to be the primary source of such infections.[28] Even in patients with malignancies (who have higher clostridial infection rates than other patients), the intestinal tract is usually the source—due to mucosal ulceration secondary to tumor invasion or chemotherapy.[90] Trauma to the intestinal tract as minimal as a barium enema has been implicated in causing infections.[505] Although *C perfringens* sepsis is a devastating infection, occasionally *C perfringens* is grown in blood cultures from patients who are not particularly ill. As many as 20% of inpatients may have skin carriage in their antecubital fossae—particularly the elderly and very ill patients with prolonged hospitalization.[5] This, together with the resistance of clostridial spores to the usual skin disinfectants,[5, 28] may account for occasional *C perfringens* as contaminants in blood cultures. *C perfringens* has been isolated from many other nosocomially infected sites, such as empyemas and necrotizing pneumonias.[48] It is frequently cultured from postoperative abdominal wound infections in mixtures with other microbes, and its pathogenic role in such situations is not clear.

Though not a true infection, another form of disease, caused by *C perfringens* is food poisoning. This is usually caused by ingestion of food containing preformed enterotoxin by *C perfringens* that has been allowed to replicate in the food. Onset usually occurs 10 to 24 hours after ingesting the toxin, and symptoms consist of primarily crampy abdominal pain and diarrhea—usually lasting less than 24 hours. A nosocomial outbreak of *C perfringens* food poisoning was recently reported to involve at least 46 patients.[607] It is probable that such occurrences are more common than is generally recognized.

Clostridium septicum

An anaerobic gram-positive, spore-forming bacillus, this organism has a normal habitat that appears to be the intestinal tract of humans and animals. Pure infections with this organism are relatively uncommon. In recent years several studies have shown a strong correlation between *C septicum* infection, especially septicemia, and underlying malignant disease—most often leukemia.[12, 355] Gastrointestinal tract lesions appear to be the source of the organisms.

Clostridium tetani

This is another anaerobic, gram-positive, spore-forming bacillus. As with other species of the genus, its spores are ubiquitous in the environment, and the vegetative forms are normal inhabitants of the intestinal tract. Nosocomial tetanus is virtually limited to neonatal tetanus, which accounts for approximately 10% of all tetanus cases in the United States.[344] Neonatal tetanus usually is due to umbilical infections acquired during birth. In most instances infections occur in infants whose mothers are not immunized to tetanus and come from lower socioeconomic populations. Person-to-person spread is not a problem.

Clostridium species

These are anaerobic, gram-positive, spore-forming bacilli. Numerous other clostridial species occur as bowel flora and occasionally cause nosocomial infections. These include cases of bacteremia and sepsis.[13, 237, 496, 667]

Not all blood cultures that are positive for *Clostridium* species are significant, and such findings must be interpreted in light of the clinical picture. When significant, the patient is often severely ill. Underlying predisposing factors to these infections include intra-abdominal disorders[13] and neoplasms.[13, 498, 667] The bowel is the presumed source.

A recent report has implicated *C butyricum* as the etiologic agent of neonatal necrotizing enterocolitis.[283] To date this has not been confirmed. If it is true, however, it will open the door to an understanding of the pathogenesis and provide rational approaches to the management of this extremely serious neonatal disease.

Coronavirus

This group of viruses commonly causes upper respiratory infections in humans.[294] It has been documented as the cause of family outbreaks of respiratory illness, but to date nosocomial infections have not been reported, although they undoubtedly occur.

Corynebacterium diphtheriae

Toxigenic strains of this gram-positive, catalase-positive, nonmotile, facultative bacillus are bona fide pathogens. Despite widespread immunization against diphtheria, occasional cases and outbreaks still occur. Nosocomial outbreaks have been reported, primarily in mental hospitals.[20, 243] The disease is contagious, and infected patients should be isolated and cared for by immunized personnel. Immunization protects against the disease diphtheria but does not protect against the carrier state; ie, immunized persons may be or become carriers. The cutaneous form of the disease is more contagious than the usual pharyngeal form.[54, 335]

Corynebacterium species

These are gram-positive, usually catalase-positive and nonmotile aerobic or facultative coryneform bacilli. These so-called diphtheroids are common components of human flora of the skin, upper respiratory tract, gastrointestinal tract, and genitourinary tract. Although their isolation from clinical material is common and almost always insignificant, bona fide infections, including nosocomial infections, have been documented. These have included systemic infections,[312, 485, 643] wound infections,[312] endocarditis involving prosthetic valves,[225, 302] and meningitis.[312] The species are commonly isolated from infected burns,[572] but their pathogenic role here is not apparent. There have been two recent reports of an unusual *Corynebacterium* species producing serious infections in oncology patients.[261, 464] This species, as yet unnamed, tends to produce a green sheen on blood agar plates and is resistant to most antimicrobics. In addition to underlying malignancy, other predisposing conditions for this infection appear to be long hospitalization, preliminary colonization, prolonged neutropenia, and previous antimicrobic therapy. The source of this species and its general epidemiology are still poorly understood. Nondiphtheria corynebacterial infections usually are considered to be of endogenous origin.

Coxsackieviruses

Members of the enteroviruses, these viruses are most often found in the gastrointestinal tract but are recognized causes of infections outside the alimentary canal, often in epidemic proportions. Such infections have included "aseptic" meningitis, myocarditis, pleuritis, and cutaneous eruptions. Although community epidemics are the rule, nosocomial outbreaks have been reported, eg, an outbreak of hand, foot, and mouth disease due to coxsackie A9 in a hospital ward[285] and an outbreak of coxsackie B5 meningitis in a newborn intensive care unit, which occurred during a community outbreak,[597] as well as other nursery outbreaks.[293, 296] Isolation of such infected patients is recommended, although its value is not certain.

Creutzfeldt-Jakob disease virus

Creutzfeldt-Jakob syndrome is presenile dementing illness caused by a virus. The natural mode of transmission and the incubation period are not known. Recent reports of nosocomial transmission of this disease have caused considerable concern among physicians and hospital personnel. In one instance, the transmission was via a corneal transplant;[160] in another, accidental inoculation of two neurosurgical patients occurred during surgery via stereotactic electrodes contaminated by a previous patient who had the illness.[63] The incubation period in these cases was 15 to 20 months. Adding to the concern is the resistance of the virus to inactivation by agents such as 70% alcohol and 10% formalin. However, it is inactivated by phenolics, iodophors, and 5% hypochlorite, as well as autoclaving for one hour at 121 C and 20 psi. The virus has been isolated from virtually all organs of infected individuals—though in far fewer numbers in other organs than in the central nervous system. The illness is relatively uncommon, afflicting 200 to 300 persons in the United States annually. Measurable increased risk of infection for hospital personnel has not been documented epidemiologically. Possible exceptions may be personnel working in the areas of neurosurgery and ophthalmologic surgery. General precautions regarding patients in these areas should include the following:

1. Needles and needle electrodes should be autoclaved and, if possible, discarded.
2. Contaminated equipment (eg, catheters, manometers, and cerebrospinal fluid counting chambers) should be decontaminated with an iodophor, phenolic or 5% hypochlorite.
3. Superficial (cutaneous) contamination of personnel by patient secretions or excretions should be treated by thorough washing with soap and water. The same applies to blood and cerebrospinal fluid contamination.
4. Accidental needle sticks or other percutaneous exposure to contaminated material should be managed by thorough cleansing of the wound with an iodophor, phenolic or 0.5% hypochlorite.
5. Special isolation is not required.
6. Demented or confused patients should not be accepted for blood or organ donations.

For a more detailed and complete listing of precautions recommended in treating this illness, the reader is referred to Gajdusek et al.[214]

Cryptococcus neoformans

In contrast to *Candida* species, this encapsulated yeast is not an endogenous human organism. It has been isolated from barnyard soil and is frequently found in pigeon excreta. Human infections are primarily pulmonary and presumably acquired by inhalation of airborne yeast cells. The primary infection is often asymptomatic and nonprogressive; it either resolves spontaneously or remains latent. In a small percentage of cases, the infection progresses to involve other organs. It has a predilection for the CNS but may become systemic. Patients with malignancies, particularly those with leukemia or lymphoma, are especially susceptible to disseminated cryptococcosis, usually with CNS involvement. This illness is associated with high mortality and poor response to amphotericin B. Characteristically, the primary disease is far advanced when the infection occurs, with the patients being leukopenic and lymphopenic and usually receiving corticosteroids.[313] There is no evidence of person-to-person communicability.

Cunninghamella elegans

Though found in nature, this phycomycete is an uncommon cause of disease in humans. Infections may occur in severely debilitated patients; eg, a fatal pulmonary infection in a patient with chronic myelocytic leukemia was apparently a nosocomial infection.[342]

Curvularia species

The species is a common saprophytic mold, often isolated as a laboratory contaminant. It has been documented as a cause of endocarditis involving a porcine aortic valve graft, presumably due to contamination of the valve prior to or at the time of insertion.[323]

Cytomegalovirus

This virus belongs to the herpesvirus group. It is a common infecting agent of humans—as manifested by the fact that 70%–100% of adults in various geographic regions have experienced cytomegalovirus (CMV) infection (blood or serologic studies).[428, 646] Many infections are undoubtedly subclinical. The mechanisms of infection include: (1) neonatal via transplacental transmission of CMV from mother to infant, (2) perinatal via infant acquisition of CMV from the birth canal of an infected mother, (3) contact with excretions of infected person, (4) iatrogenic via transfusion or allografts from infected persons,[95, 309, 488, 596, 612] and (5) reactivation of latent CMV infections due to altered host–parasite relationships.[193, 410, 428, 596] Although considerable controversy has existed regarding the latter two mechanisms of active disease, it now appears clear that both mechanisms do occur and together constitute the most frequent means of nosocomial active CMV infection. In the case of blood transfusions, infected leukocytes appear to be primarily responsible for the transmission of CMV infections, since the transfusion of deglycerolized frozen blood (essentially leukocyte-free) to seronegative recipients does not result in seroconversion.[612] The average incubation period is about eight weeks. The clinical manifestations of CMV infection are legion and varied. They include CMV mononucleosis, postperfusion syndrome, interstitial pneumonitis, hepatitis, fever, arthralgia, leukopenia, retinitis, hepatosplenomegaly, and myalgia. Predisposing conditions and precipitating events that are particularly associated with CMV infection include leukemia,[273, 377, 518] lymphomas,[345, 377, 518] bone marrow transplants (particularly prone to CMV interstitial pneumonitis),[273, 404, 437] renal allografts,[193, 428, 596] postperfusion syndrome following cardiac surgery,[95, 310, 496] and posttransfusion hepatitis.[488] Some form of immunosuppression appears to be a significant contributory factor in many instances.

The diagnosis of CMV infections is based on serologic tests, culture examination, and/or cytologic or histologic identification of diagnostic intranuclear inclusion bodies—in order of decreasing sensitivity. None of these tests provides a truly practical routine approach to the early diagnosis of CMV infection in the average hospital. Most diagnoses of CMV infections are therefore based on clinical impressions, which may be retrospectively confirmed by serologic studies. This renders ongoing surveillance of nosocomial CMV infections difficult and, for the average institution, impractical. However, for institutions with large numbers of high-risk patients, some attempt at surveillance is encouraged. Two recent studies showed that patients who developed primary CMV infections had a greater risk of developing suprainfections by bacterial and fungal agents.[119,496] This adds an additional dimension to the significance of CMV infections.

Proven means of preventing nosocomial CMV infections are not currently available. The prevention of reactivation of a latent CMV infection is a particularly difficult problem. The prophylaxis of primary CMV infection, however, remains theoretically attainable with current knowledge. Such attempts should be directed toward high-risk patients who have negative CMV serology. CMV-negative candidates for renal or bone marrow transplants should, when possible, receive tissue from CMV-negative donors. Since CMV is shed in various excretions (eg, urine and saliva) for varying periods of time by infected persons, it may be reasonable to isolate patients with suspected or known CMV infection from high-risk susceptible patients.

Desulfovibrio species

Anaerobic vibrio-like, gram-negative bacilli, members of this genus may be found in part of the normal colonic flora and are of extremely low pathogenicity. One case report of nosocomial *D desulfuricans* bacteremia has been published,[484] but its clinical significance is questionable.

Epstein-Barr virus

This virus belongs to the herpesvirus group. As with other herpesviruses, human experience with Epstein-Barr virus (EBV) is almost universal. By the age of 30, 80%–100% of people have serologic evidence of previous EBV infection. Most often this is manifested clinically as infectious mononucleosis and occurs primarily in adolescents. In members of lower socioeconomic groups, infections tend to occur earlier in childhood, often with atypical manifestations.[272] EBV may be isolated from actively infected patients from lymphocytes and throat and salivary secretions and may persist for years.[117,272,436,592] Subclinical reactivated EBV infections are probably not uncommon in normal adults,[593] and as many as 16% of clinically normal adults may yield positive EBV cultures from throat washings.[117] However, this percentage is significantly higher in patients with renal grafts,[117,428,592] drug-induced immunosuppression,[592] acute lymphocytic leukemia,[117] non-Hodgkin's lymphoma,[117] plasma cell myeloma, and acute and chronic myelocytic leukemia.[117] In addition to its association with many malignancies, EBV has been implicated etiologically in certain malignancies such as Burkitt's lymphoma and nasopharyngeal carcinoma.[172, 406] The occasional cases of acute lymphocytic leukemia that closely follow infectious mononucleosis suggest a possible etiologic relationship.[359] The forms of EBV infection in humans take on a rather complex pattern, which can be summarized as follows[172]: EBV infections may be productive (virus replication with cell death, eg, infectious mononucleosis) or nonproductive (virus genome present within the cell). Productive infections may be primary or secondary (reactivated). Nonproductive infections may be expressed (malignant transformation) or unexpressed. Unexpressed nonproductive infections may become activated to productive infections by an alteration in the host–parasite relationship.

Most active nosocomial EBV infections fall into the last category. However, true primary EBV or EBV reinfection occasionally may be nosocomial. Examples include a case of transmission of EBV infection by plasma transfusion[620] and an outbreak of HB-negative hepatitis in a dialysis unit.[131] In the latter instance, 11 of 40 patients in a hemodialysis unit developed HBAg-negative hepatitis during a five-week period. Ten of these had serologic evidence of recent EBV infection and had used the same venous pressure monitor, in which evidence of blood reflux was found—indicating the probable means of transmission.

Despite the presence of EBV in the blood and salivary secretions of actively infected patients, person-to-person transmission appears to require close and usually prolonged contact. Consequently, isolation of such patients does not seem to be routinely warranted, except possibly from patients at high risk.

Echoviruses

These members of the enteroviruses are commonly isolated from the intestinal tract, but infections of other sites also occur, such as exanthems and respiratory tract and CNS infections. Although these are generally considered to be community-acquired infections, they probably occur nosocomially with greater frequency than is recognized—as suggested by the recent report of an outbreak in a special-care baby unit in which nine infants were infected with echovirus 11 and three of them died,[423] as well as other nursery outbreaks.[293, 296] Isolation is recommended, but more extreme measures may be necessary to end outbreaks.

Edwardsiella tarda

This gram-negative, facultative, fermentative bacillus belongs to the family Enterobacteriaceae. The exact pathogenic status of this species is not fully known. It appears to be a potential enteric pathogen, producing symptoms from mild diarrhea to severe gastroenteritis with fever, vomiting, and watery diarrhea, especially in the very young and the aged.[70] A carrier state exists, but its frequency is not known. Nosocomial infections do occur and are not limited to gastroenteritis, eg, postoperative wound infections.[305] Its potential spectrum is probably comparable with that of other Enterobacteriaceae, but to date it is much less frequently encountered. Patients with *E tarda* enteritis should be in enteric isolation.

Eikenella corrodens

This is a gram-negative, nonfermentative, nonoxidative, oxidase-positive bacillus. This organism is a recently recognized potential human pathogen, and its normal ecology has not yet been elucidated fully. It appears to be a normal inhabitant of the oropharynx[674, 675] and probably of the gastrointestinal tract. Both community-acquired and nosocomial infections have been caused by *Eikenella corrodens*, either alone or in combination with other organisms.[155, 674, 675]

Documented infections have included endocarditis, meningitis, empyema, wound infections, and abscesses. Predisposing factors so far recognized are advanced age, underlying malignancy, and ruptured viscus.[155]

Entamoeba histolytica

An amebic intestinal parasite, this is the major cause of the disease known as amebic dysentery. Infection is acquired by ingestion of the cyst form. Although outbreaks have been traced to common sources such as contaminated water supplies, the most common means of spread is person to person via the fecal-oral route. Nosocomial outbreaks have been reported,[338, 551] and they are more likely to occur in health care facilities for long-term care such as mental hospitals than in acute care community hospitals.

Enterobacter species

These are facultative, fermentative, gram-negative bacilli belonging to the family Enterobacteriaceae. The three major species commonly encountered in clinical specimens are *E cloacae*, *E aerogenes*, and *E agglomerans*. (*E gergoviae* and *E sakazaki* are names suggested by the CDC for biotypic variants of the first two.) *Enterobacter* species commonly inhabit the human intestinal tract but rarely in large numbers. Members of this genus are common nosocomial pathogens, readily colonize other parts of the body in hospitalized patients, and often cause infections of the urinary tract, respiratory tract, and wounds.[476, 516] Isolated and sporadic infections are usually endogenous and not readily communicable. Outbreaks, on the other hand, are often due to contaminated exogenous sources. Examples of such sources are contaminated intravenous fluids,[105, 400] contaminated blood transfusions,[189] contaminated platelet products,[80] ice from an improperly plumbed, contaminated ice machine,[437] and contaminated urinals.[419] A national outbreak occurred recently and was traced to contaminated inner cap assemblies of commercial intravenous fluid bottles.[98] Many infections, particularly those of *E cloacae*, are serious and may lead to sepsis and death.[516] The potential sources and types of infection caused by the genus *Enterobacter* are virtually unlimited.

Enterobacteriaceae

This is the name of a large family of gram-negative bacilli that as a group are facultative, oxidase-negative glucose fermenters. Its members are commonly cultured from the intestinal tract either as normal inhabitants or as true enteric pathogens. Normally colonization of sites other than the intestinal tract by Enterobacteriaceae is uncommon and transient. In hospitalized patients, this does not seem to be the case. The incidence of pharyngeal colonization, for example, is significantly higher in hospitalized patients, and the incidence of such colonization correlates best with the severity of patient disease.[299] Antimicrobic therapy, inhalation therapy, and duration of hospitalization seem to play minor (if any) roles. Pharyngeal colonization by Enterobacteriaceae in hospital personnel who have patient contact is no different from that in other personnel.[493] The mechanism of Enterobacteriaceae colonization of the pharynx and other sites of debilitated patients is poorly understood. Such colonization, however, appears to be an important first step in the pathogenesis of infection in these patients, particularly in cases of pneumonia.[299, 300, 440] Enterobacteriaceae are readily transferred from person to person via hands, and the best prophylaxis against this is frequent hand-washing. Depending on the organism and type of infection, isolation may or may not be appropriate.

Escherichia coli

This facultative gram-negative bacillus belongs to the family Enterobacteriaceae. It is a normal inhabitant of the intestinal tract and is, in fact, the most prevalent Enterobacteriaceae species normally found there. Yet its presence in the intestinal tract is not always benign. *E coli* is clearly a major cause of gastroenteritis and has been responsible for a significant number of nosocomial outbreaks.[216, 327, 357, 624] These are usually due to enteroinvasive (*Shigella*-like) strains or enterotoxigenic strains.[216] Two types of toxins have so far been identified: a heat-stable toxin and a cholera-like, heat-labile toxin. There is also a colonization factor (K antigen) that may be important in pathogenesis. Many, if not all, of these enteropathogenic characteristics of *E coli* are plasmid-mediated. There are still some *E coli* gastroenteritis outbreaks in which none of the recognized enteropathogenic factors has been found,[357] indicating that other mechanisms also exist. Although these enteropathogenic factors are clearly associated with enteric infections, there is no correlation between the presence of these factors and *E coli* infections at other sites.[631] Parenthetically, it should be noted that routine serotyping for the classical enteropathogenic *E coli* serotypes is of little or no value in solitary cases, but may be of value in outbreak situations.[216]

E coli is the number one nosocomial pathogen and accounts for nearly a third of all bacterial nosocomial infections, the majority of which are urinary tract infections (see Table 3–1). In addition, however, it is a significant nosocomial pathogen in other infections such as postoperative wound infection (see Table 5–1), respiratory infection (see Table 4–1),[610] septicemia (see Table 7–2),[512] endocarditis,[585] and neonatal meningitis.[391, 511, 512, 532, 659] Underlying conditions that increase the prevalence of infections generally (eg, diabetes mellitus and malignancies) also predispose to *E coli* infections.[580] Of interest is the apparent predilection of *E coli* infections for patients with sickle cell disease.[512]

Despite the voluminous literature on *E coli*, the epidemiology and pathogenesis of nosocomial *E coli* infections are not fully understood, although much is surmised. Many nosocomial *E coli* infections clearly are caused by endogenous *E coli* with which patients were colonized at the time of admission,[62, 618] whereas others are caused by *E coli* acquired after admission to the hospital. It is now believed that food may be a major source of nosocomial *E coli* colonization of the intestinal tract.[129, 275, 557] Strains of *E coli* have been traced from slaughtered animals to abattoirs, to hospital kitchens, to hospital food, and to fecal flora of patients.[532] Although *E coli* is normally a prevalent facultative component of the intestinal flora, the prevalent strains or types are in constant flux,[618] and the duration of colonization of the colon by ingested strains may vary from 1 to more than 300 days.[129] Aside from the association of the K-1 antigen with central nervous system invasiveness in neonates,[391, 511, 532] microbial virulence factors of *E coli* in nonenteric infections are virtually unknown or at best poorly understood.

Because of the frequency of nosocomial infections caused by *E coli*, common source outbreaks are often difficult to detect without some means of strain or type identification. Methods of typing that have been found epidemiologically useful include serotyping,[129, 327, 528, 557, 580, 618] colicin typing,[129, 275] resistogram typing,[169] and biotyping.[212] Biotyping is particularly useful as a screening tool since it can be incorporated simultaneously into the identification procedure.[212]

Flavobacterium species

These are oxidase-positive, indole-positive, oxidative, gram-negative bacilli. Members of this genus are common inhabitants of moist areas in the environment, and in hospitals are often cultured from sinks and various items containing water or saline. *Flavobacterium* species may be resistant to chlorine in water in concentrations as high as 0.6 to 3.0 ppm[274] and to aqueous chlorhexidine (1:1,000).[132] The species most often implicated in nosocomial infections has been *F meningosepticum*. Though not usually considered a component of human microbial flora, this species was isolated 88 times from 27,600 genitourinary cultures, for a carriage rate of 0.3%.[447] It is postulated that such colonization may be the source of sporadic cases of neonatal meningitis due to *F meningosepticum* in which environmental sources cannot be found. Outbreaks of neonatal meningitis are one of the major problems caused by this organism,[267, 380, 479] but infections in adults such as septicemia[446, 583] and pneumonia[601] also are being reported with increasing frequency. In most outbreaks an environmental source usually can be found, such as contaminated saline used for neonatal eye wash,[479] contaminated anesthetic vials,[446] contaminated multiple-dose drug vials,[445] and contaminated ice for cooling syringes used in arterial catheters.[583] In one neonatal intensive care unit, two *F meningosepticum* outbreaks occurred in which upper respiratory tract colonization preceded infection.[267] *Flavobacterium* species other than *F meningosepticum* occasionally cause infections but are usually contaminants.[583]

Fusarium moniliforme

This species is a saprophytic mold and common laboratory contaminant. It may rarely cause infections in severely debilitated and immunosuppressed patients; eg, systemic *Fusarium* infection has been found in denuded skin following varicella zoster in a lymphoma patient who was receiving steroids and chemotherapy.[670]

Geotrichum candidum

This fungus is characterized by both blastospore and arthrospore formation. It may be found among the normal flora of the upper respiratory tract, intestinal tract, and genitourinary tract. Infections by this organism are rare and usually occur in debilitated patients; eg, geotrichosis with fungemia occurred in a patient who had bronchogenic carcinoma.[227]

Hafnia alvei

Also called *Enterobacter hafniae*, this fermentative, gram-negative bacillus belongs to the family Enterobacteriaceae. This organism is presumably a normal component of human fecal flora but is present in relatively small numbers. Although nosocomial infections by *H alvei* do occur,[171, 639] their frequency is low compared with that of infections caused by other Enterobacteriaceae. Infections include sepsis, abscesses, and respiratory tract and wound infections. In the period 1975–1977, we encountered three such infections—two respiratory tract infections and one septicemia with no known primary site.

Hemophilus aphrophilus

This small gram-negative bacillus usually requires carbon dioxide and heme for primary isolation. It is a normal component of the upper respiratory tract flora. *H aphrophilus* infections are relatively rare, but bacterial endocarditis and brain abscess account for more than half of such reported infections.[64, 336, 452] We have seen only one case of *H aphrophilis* infection, an endocarditis involving a Starr-Edwards prosthetic mitral valve. Nosocomial postoperative wound infections with this organism have been reported in most large studies. It may be more prevalent than generally appreciated because of its fastidiousness on primary isolation, and it may be overgrown easily in mixed cultures.

Hemophilus influenzae and H parainfluenzae

These organisms are small, fastidious, gram-negative bacilli, which are commonly cultured from the upper respiratory tract of normal individuals. Infections are most often due to the encapsulated type of *H influenzae* and occur most often in infants and in the elderly—particularly those with chronic obstructive pulmonary disease. Meningitis and sepsis are the serious forms of *Hemophilus* infection in infants and usually occur in infants older than two months, when maternal antibodies have largely disappeared. There have been reports of nosocomial neonatal infections both by *H influenzae*[240, 328] and by *H parainfluenzae*.[254] Although less than 1% of normal and pregnant women have cervical colonization by these organisms, there is evidence that neonatal infections are caused by *Hemophilus* species acquired during transit of the infant through the colonized birth canal.[328] In our own experience, nosocomial *H influenzae* infections have occurred most often in elderly patients with advanced chronic obstructive pulmonary disease. In these cases the source appears to be organisms harbored by the patients at the time of admission. This organism accounts for 6.2% of the nosocomial respiratory tract infections in our institution (see Table 4–1). There has been no evidence of nosocomial cross-infections.

Hemophilus vaginalis

This gram-variable bacillus is also known as *Corynebacterium vaginale*, and its taxonomic status is presently unsettled. It has been a difficult microbe to assess microbiologically, epidemiologically, and clinically. Approximately a third of normal asymptomatic women have vaginal colonization by *H vaginalis*. Colonization is more prevalent in nonwhites, users of birth control pills, and women who have never been married or pregnant.[389] There has been considerable controversy over its possible role in vaginitis. However, occasional serious bona fide infections have been documented as caused by this agent. In a case of puerperal sepsis in an 18-year-old woman 24 hours after a cesarian section, *H vaginalis* was cultured from blood and endometrium.[500] In the past few years we have seen several cases of nosocomial UTIs due to this organism.

Characteristically, patients who had UTIs due to *H vaginalis* were catheterized, had typical UTI signs and symptoms, and yielded *H vaginalis* in quantities greater than 10^5/ml in pure urine culture. In most instances urine cultures became negative within 48 hours after removal of the catheter, but in at least two instances antimicrobic therapy was required. Although *H vaginalis* infections are rarely serious, we believe they are more common than generally suspected. This may be due in part to the inadequacy of many "routine" culture methods in detecting these organisms.

Hepatitis A virus

This is the viral agent that causes so-called hepatitis A (HA). Based on seroepidemiologic studies and reviews,[142, 148, 152] hepatitis A virus (HAV) is widespread in the human population, with as many as 80% of adults showing serologic evidence of previous experience with this agent. The incidence increases with age and with decreasing socioeconomic status and poor hygiene. Transmission of HAV from person to person occurs primarily by the fecal-oral route. Following infection there is a two- to six-week incubation period during which the patient is asymptomatic. Toward the end of this period, there develops a viremia with extensive fecal shedding of the virus. Shortly after the onset of clinical symptoms of hepatitis (if they develop), viremia and viral shedding cease—usually before peak enzyme levels are reached.[147, 494] It is during this shedding period that the disease is infectious, particularly before clinical symptoms develop since precautions are less likely to be taken during that time. A carrier status for HAV is not currently recognized. The clinical illness of HA is variable but is usually mild and only very rarely progresses to chronic active hepatitis. Blood donated by a person who is in the asymptomatic viremic stage is a theoretical source of transfusion hepatitis, but this must be extremely rare in reality. Such a source has been implicated in a couple of reports.[92, 402] Foodborne outbreaks of HA, including nosocomial outbreaks, have been well documented and usually can be traced to an infected food-preparer.[403]

Current evidence indicates that patients with HA are no longer infectious once their enzyme levels have peaked, and consequently the standard enteric isolation and precautions are not necessary after this stage of the disease. The problem, however, rests with our current inability to make an unequivocal diagnosis of HA. Currently available methods allow us to only rule hepatitis B in or out. Non-A, non-B hepatitis cannot be reliably differentiated clinically from HA. Although methods for the serodiagnosis of HA soon will be approved, until then it should be assumed that these cases are not HA, and patients should be isolated accordingly.

Hepatitis B virus

This viral agent causes hepatitis B (HB)—the classic transfusion hepatitis. Recent years have brought huge advances in our understanding of HB and HBV, but many questions are still unanswered. The primary means of transmission of HB is the parenteral introduction of infected blood. The ability to detect HBV surface antigen (HB_sAg) and antibody (HB_sAb), the application of such tests by blood banks to all donated blood, and the removal of blood that is positive for HB_sAg have drastically reduced the incidence of transfusion HB.[15] On the other hand, the ability to detect HB_sAg has led to a number of epidemiologic problems previously unforeseen.

Typically, in cases of HB there is an incubation period of two to six months following inoculation of HBV during which the patient is asymptomatic. As with HA, the viremic stage begins toward the end of the incubation period, but unlike HA, the viremia in HB may persist for much longer periods. Those who are viremic beyond the period of clinical illness are referred to as *carriers*, and this state may persist for years. In studying both HB patients and HBV carriers, it was found that unlike HA, HB_sAg was not commonly shed in feces.[609] On the other hand, it was found frequently in saliva,[268, 628, 636] nasal washings,[609] urine,[609] vaginal secretions, sweat,[600] semen,[268] and amniotic fluid.[387] If HB_sAg correlates with infectivity, these findings suggest that the nonparenteral potential for HB transmission should be high. In fact, however, with a few exceptions, most epidemiologic studies suggest that the nonparenteral transmission of HB is probably quite rare.[14, 364, 405] The highest rates of nosocomial HB currently occur in patients in renal dialysis units,[221, 297, 370, 576, 662] but the potential for contact with contaminated or infected blood is high and is a more likely explanation than contact with secretions. The same is true for the higher incidence seen in some laboratories[662] as well as the fact that many commercially prepared control sera may be contaminated.[650] The institution of control measures in England has apparently reduced this risk significantly in laboratories.[250] In nosocomial outbreaks that can be traced to a particular patient, the potential for a blood source is apparent in some[522] but not all.[79] Oncology patients may have a higher carrier rate than the normal population,[594] and at least one outbreak in an oncology ward has been reported that has no obvious blood contamination.[635] The overall incidence of HB_sAg and HB_sAb in hospital personnel is higher than that in the general population,[361] but this difference can be accounted for in large part by those employees (dialysis personnel, operating room personnel, etc) who are most likely to come in contact with blood.[297] It would appear, therefore, that body secretions or fluids other than blood occasionally may be the source of HBV infections, but the most common source is blood via the inapparent parenteral route.

The recently discovered E antigen of HBV has been shown to correlate with the presence of DNA polymerase.[16] Furthermore, there is a strong correlation between the presence of E antigen in HB_sAg-positive patients and infectivity.[16, 554] If such a correlation is substantiated, E antigen testing will be a most valuable aid in determining the disposition of HB_sAg-positive patients and hospital personnel.

From the infection control standpoint, the approach to the management of persons with HB is based on concepts that are likely to continue to change. The recommendations of Snydman et al should be familiar to all involved in this area.[574] Routine HB_sAg testing of personnel and patients is not generally recommended except for those in high-risk areas such as dialysis units. Most important, perhaps, is for infection control personnel to be constantly aware of new information in this area as it becomes available and to constantly and extensively review and alter, when indicated, their own control measures.

Hepatitis non-A, non-B virus

An outgrowth of the many advances in our knowledge of HA and HB has been the recognition that there are still many cases of viral hepatitis that are not due to HAV or HBV.[146, 183, 282, 401, 487] Some of these may be due to other known viruses, such as cytomegalovirus,[183] but most appear to be due to an agent (or agents) as yet unidentified. These cases have been variously designated hepatitis C or hepatitis non-A, non-B. Since some outbreaks have had short incubation periods that resemble those of HA[401] and others have long incubation periods resembling those of HB,[487] it is possible that more than one agent is responsible for hepatitis non-A, non-B. A recent report describes the presence of a non-A, non-B antigen (referred to as HC antigen) in the acute sera from 13 of 13 patients with the long incubation form and from 4 of 10 with the short incubation form.[555] Since the epidemiology and infectivity of non-A, non-B hepatitis are not yet known, it is best for hospital infection control programs to be conservative in the disposition of such cases; ie, enteric and needle precautions should be used.

Herpes simplex virus

Herpesvirus hominis is a large viral agent belonging to the herpesvirus group. Herpes simplex virus (HSV) is widespread in the human population, with virtually 100% of adults having experienced infection by it. Following a primary HSV infection, the virus has the capacity to remain latent (or dormant) in nerve ganglia (eg, the trigeminal ganglion). Stressful stimuli may reactivate the virus, converting the asymptomatic latent infection into an active symptomatic one again. In the majority of people this amounts to a relatively minor, though quite annoying, herpes labialis or one of its variants. There are two major antigenic variants of HSV, type 1 and type 2, that characteristically cause herpes labialis and herpes progenitalis, respectively; however, this is only a rule of thumb and many exceptions occur.

Two major forms of nosocomial HSV infections merit brief discussion here: neonatal and postnatal. Neonatal infections are relatively uncommon. Although transplacental infection may occur from viremic mothers and is manifest by clinical disease of the infant at birth or within the first two days of life,[263] this is much less common than acquisition of the infection while the infant is passing through the HSV-infected birth canal.[263, 284, 651] Most neonatal infections are due to HSV type 2 and may vary in severity from minor vesicular lesions to severe disseminated lesions and encephalitis.[570] Herpes progenitalis is up to three times more common in pregnant women, and as many as 1% of pregnant women in lower socioeconomic populations may be infected.[263] The incidence increases with the progression of pregnancy. The risk of neonatal infection is about 10% in women who have herpes progenitalis after 32 weeks of gestation, and if lesions are present at the time of delivery, the risk is estimated to be about 40% if the infant is delivered per vaginum. Some studies suggest the risk is much lower, however.[529] Nevertheless, there appears to be general agreement that when women have active genital HSV infection at the time of delivery, the infant should be delivered by cesarean section whenever possible. The effectiveness of this prophylactic measure, though theoretically sound, has not been proved. There is at least one report of an infant with neonatal disseminated HSV infection despite cesarean-section delivery, but in this instance rupture of the membranes occurred 12 hours prior to the cesarean section.[425] Infected infants should be isolated. Outbreaks of HSV infection in a nursery may occur via indirect spread through hospital personnel from an index case.[207] Although there is no good documentation that personnel with active herpetic lesions are a significant source of nosocomial HSV infections, it may be prudent for such personnel to refrain from attending to high-risk patients such as neonates.

Postnatal nosocomial HSV infections are usually (but not always) reactivated infections that occur as a result of a specific stimulus or significant immunosuppression or both. The classic example of the former is a study of 56 patients, otherwise normal, who underwent trigeminal nerve root decompression for trigeminal neuralgia, of whom 50% developed reactivated HSV infection.[461] HSV infections related to immunosuppression fall into two major groups. First are those patients with malignancies, whose disease as well as their therapy renders them immunosuppressed.[418, 519] Clinically HSV infections in such patients often are atypical (and hence often missed); the most common infections are mucocutaneous or esophageal but not uncommon may be disseminated infections with involvement of lungs, liver, and other organs. The second major group of patients are organ transplant recipients, who are usually subjected to marked immunosuppressive therapy to avoid transplant rejection. These patients are particularly susceptible to HSV infection during the first three months after the transplantation. This propensity has been described for renal transplants,[412, 427, 428] cardiac transplants,[497] and lung transplants.[157] Infection appears to be associated with defective cellular immunity (despite normal antibody production), which returns to normal after three months.[497] Another clinical setting for nosocomial HSV infection that may be more common than is currently appreciated is the burn patient.[199] Serious HSV infections of burns are documented and may be a significant predisposing factor to secondary bacterial infections and sepsis.

Although the majority of postnatal nosocomial HSV infections in the settings described above are probably due to reactivation of latent virus, reinfections and primary infections have been shown to occur, with outbreaks resulting from person-to-person transfer through personnel.[81, 461] Differentiation of a common strain outbreak from multiple cases of reactivated infection requires good epidemiologic investigations with documentation of a common strain. Although some methods for this are described and found to be usable,[81] such methods are not practical for the average clinical laboratory.

Histoplasma capsulatum

This is a dimorphic fungus pathogenic for humans. Primary infections by this agent are almost invariably community-acquired; however, recrudescent or reactivated infections may occur in previously infected individuals who are subjected to immunosuppression.[150]

Influenza viruses

These viral agents cause influenza. Influenza is a seasonal respiratory infection that often occurs in epidemic and pandemic proportions. Nosocomial outbreaks also occur, usually in association with community outbreaks. The period of infectivity is from as early as two days before the onset of symptoms to about three days afterward. There is no evidence that routine isolation of such patients is effective in controlling the spread of such infections, and consequently it is not generally recommended.[280] Vaccination should be available for hospital personnel during epidemic periods.

In addition to its own morbidity, influenza virus infections also may predispose infected patients to superimposed bacterial pneumonia.[542] This is often due to *Staphylococcus aureus*, is found commonly in the elderly and those with chronic pulmonary disease, and is associated with significant mortality.

Klebsiella pneumoniae

This facultative gram-negative bacillus belongs to the family Enterobacteriaceae. Two common biotypes are often given species status: *K ozenae* and *K oxytoca*. We have been unable to appreciate any significant epidemiologic differences among these, but such differentiation is useful in the investigation of *Klebsiella* species infection outbreaks. *K pneumoniae* is a major nosocomial pathogen, both as a cause of endogenous isolated infection and in exogenous epidemic settings. The epidemiology of *K pneumoniae* is rather complex and only partially understood. The species is a normal inhabitant of the intestinal tract. Over a period of several months, all people studied were fecal carriers of *K pneumoniae* at some time,[413] but at any given time about a third of the population (in or out of the hospital) were fecal carriers.[139] The source of such fecal colonization appears to be ingested food that contains the organism.[77, 94, 413] Although fecal carriage of *K pneumoniae* is usually asymptomatic, cases of *K pneumoniae* enteritis have been reported and may be severe.[314] Patients who become nosocomially colonized by *K pneumoniae* are more apt to develop *K pneumoniae* infection by the colonized strain.[548] Specific serotypes have been traced from the hospital kitchen to nasogastric feedings for intensive care patients, to fecal flora of patients ingesting these contaminated feedings, to clinical infections in colonized patients as well as other patients on the same unit.[94] Although the prevalence of nosocomial and community-acquired colonization by *K pneumoniae* is not appreciably different, the two do differ in that the frequency of multiple antibiotic resistant strains is much higher in the nosocomial group,[139, 548] which is related to the use of antibiotics.[219, 548] The antimicrobic resistance is often plasmid-mediated, but plasmid transfer to other organisms plays a minor role in outbreaks compared with colonizations by plasmid-containing organisms.[219] *K pneumoniae* is a common contaminant in the environment, and such environmental foci have been sources of *K pneumoniae* outbreaks, eg, contaminated hand cream.[417] The source of some outbreaks is never identified, although the outbreaks often are ended by control measures directed at the surroundings[641] or by discontinuation of the use of certain antimicrobics.[486] UTIs and RTIs are the most common types of nosocomial infections caused by *K pneumoniae*,[164] and together they accounted for more than 80% of the *K pneumoniae* infections in our institution. However, the spectrum of infections caused by *K pneumoniae* is large and includes meningitis, wound infections, and sepsis. In addition to the usual factors that predispose to infection in general, two epidemiologic parameters characteristically are related to nosocomial *K pneumoniae* infections: prior antimicrobic therapy[486, 548, 589, 603] and prolonged hospitalization.[385, 603]

Because of its high incidence—causing nearly 8% of nosocomial infections, the sixth most common cause—*K pneumoniae* should be typed for strain identification in investigating possible outbreaks caused by it. Practical methods for this have included biotyping, serotyping, or both.[501] Bacteriocin (Klebocin) susceptibility typing may be a valuable adjunct to other typing methods but is not yet practical for most laboratories.[83] Antimicrobic susceptibility patterns may be useful in screening efforts, but their characteristics are not stable enough to be totally reliable for typing.[672]

Lactobacillus species

These are gram-positive, asporogenous, anaerobic bacilli. Members of this genus are found among the normal flora of the gastrointestinal tract and the genitourinary tract. Although their pathogenicity is quite low, occasional infections are produced by them, including nosocomial sepsis.[46, 552] We occasionally encounter lactobacilli in pure culture in counts of greater than 10^5/ml in urine specimens, but their significance remains obscure. In most such instances, repeat culture results are equivocal or negative.

Legionella pneumophila

Legionella pneumophila (Legionnaires' disease bacilli) is a fastidious, slow-growing, gram-negative bacillus. Its ecology is under intense study currently but is not well understood. Evidence suggests that it is found in the environment and is not normally part of the human bacterial flora. It produces in humans a respiratory illness whose characteristic severe form is manifested by abrupt onset of fever, weakness, malaise, cough, and often diarrhea. Person-to-person transmission has not yet been documented. Although initial reports of Legionnaires' disease dealt with community-acquired epidemics, at least two major nosocomial outbreaks have been reported. One was a recent outbreak in a Veterans Administration hospital in California[114, 330]; the other was a 1965 outbreak in a psychiatric hospital in Washington, DC, which, retrospectively with seroepidemiologic studies, has been shown to be Legionnaires' disease.[604] In the latter outbreak, sites of recent soil excavations were implicated as the source. In the former outbreak, extensive epidemiologic studies showed only two factors that correlated significantly with the disease—prolonged hospitalization and immunosuppression. Six of 12 renal homograft recipients became infected. Because of the difficulty of culturing this organism from usual clinical specimens, the diagnosis is usually made by clinical suspicion followed by serologic confirmation.

Listeria monocytogenes

This species is a facultative, gram-positive, asporogenous, motile bacillus. This organism is apparently widespread in nature, having been isolated from soil, vegetation, and animal feces.[645, 648] It has also been shown that at least 1% of the normal population carry *L monocytogenes* in their feces, and more than 20% of contacts of patients with listeriosis carry the organism in their feces.[72] It appears that this constituent of the fecal flora is the most common source of human listeriosis and is probably ultimately derived from ingesting the organism with food. The majority of infections occur in the very young (less than 30 days of age) and the elderly (more than 50 years of age). Neonates may acquire the infection either transplacentally or during passage through the birth canal. In the former instance, infants have a disseminated granulomatous disease at the time of birth, and many are stillborn.[49, 449] Cases of habitual abortion have been attributed to this in women who have documented excretion of large numbers of *L monocytogenes* in their stools.[664] In infants who acquire the disease at the time of birth (nosocomial), two clinical forms are recognized: early onset or the septicemic form with onset in less than five days due mostly to serotypes 1a and 1b, and late onset or the meningitic form with onset usually between 10 and 20 days, due most often to serotype IVb.[10] Infection in adults is usually manifested by sepsis and/or central nervous system infection. There are several epidemiologic factors that appear to significantly predispose to infection with this organism. These include corticosteroid therapy,[301,407] organ allografts,[217,292] lymphoproliferative malignancies, [217,295,372] and splenectomies.[217,295] Such infections appear to be of endogenous origin, and the role of person-to-person transmission is not clear. One recent report of a nosocomial outbreak of *Listeria* septicemia suggested person-to-person spread, but this could not be proved.[246]

Measles virus

This large RNA virus belongs to the paramyxovirus group. It is the cause of measles, a formerly common childhood exanthem, the incidence of which has been greatly reduced by vaccines. In adults and particularly in immunosuppressed patients, infection can result in severe and even fatal illnesses.[9,396] The question has been raised as to whether such infections represent reactivation of latent virus.[9]

Micrococcus species

These are gram-positive, nonfermentative cocci. The microbes are prevalent in the environment and are a normal component of the bacterial flora of humans at various sites. Most often when cultured from clinical material, micrococci are contaminants or commensals. Nevertheless, true micrococcal infections have been documented, including nosocomial infections.[526] The differentiation between a contaminant and an infecting agent must be based on the clinical data as well as microbiologic evidence. For example, biotyping of multiple isolates of *Micrococcus* species from the blood may be useful in that multiple types suggest contamination, and identical biotypes would be more indicative of infection.

Mycobacterium tuberculosis

This acid-fast nonbranching bacterium is a primary human pathogen, the cause of tuberculosis. It may act opportunistically in the sense that reactivated secondary infections not infrequently occur in patients who are receiving immunosuppressant therapy or who are immunosuppressed because of their primary disease.[311] The organism is spread from person to person by airborne droplet nuclei. Such infectious droplets are produced by the coughing of actively infected patients, and the droplets must reach the alveolar sacs of susceptible individuals for infections to occur. In general, cross-infection requires relatively long and close contact with infected patients. The spread of infection is effectively reduced or eliminated by simple utilization of sanitary coughing procedures. The effective therapy currently available has resulted in the closing of most tuberculosis hospitals and sanataria, with the result that the disease is seen more often in general hospitals. The major problem from a nosocomial infection standpoint is the unsuspected or undiagnosed tuberculosis patients, since appropriate precautions are not taken with such patients. Such occurrences may not be uncommon and may account in part for the fact that nearly 2% of general hospital employees become infected annually—as manifested by PPD skin test conversion.[26] Under certain conditions, such as inadequate or unbalanced ventilation systems, undiagnosed patients may be the source of true nosocomial outbreaks.[167]

Mycobacterium species (atypical mycobacteria)

These are acid-fast, nonbranching bacilli. In contrast with *M tuberculosis*, atypical mycobacteria are commonly found in the environment in soil and water.[368] They are normal saprophytes of humans and animals, particularly of the oral cavity; and these organisms presumably are derived from ingested food and water.[368, 409] The pathogenicity of these species is generally less than that of *M tuberculosis*, and many species are essentially nonpathogenic. In further contrast with *M tuberculosis*, cross-infection with atypical mycobacteria does not occur, and infection by these organisms usually can be traced to an environmental source or are of endogenous origin. Atypical mycobacterial infections occur in patients with malignancies (especially head and neck carcinomas) with significantly greater frequency than in the general population.[185] Nosocomial infections caused by atypical mycobacteria are being recognized with increasing frequency. Of interest is the recent report of atypical mycobacteria (*M chelonei*) being grown from pre-implant cultures of porcine heart valves in several medical institutions and the subsequent development of infection in at least two recipients—one with culture-positive pericardial tamponade and one with an acid-fast smear-positive (culture-negative) subvalvular abscess.[107, 110] Atypical mycobacterial endocarditis in patients with prosthetic valves also has been reported.[17, 369] Outbreaks of sternal incision infections due to *M chelonei* and *M fortuitum* have been seen in patients following open heart surgery (including coronary artery as well as valvular surgery) at two hospitals.[106] Other examples of nosocomial mycobacterial infection outbreaks are abscesses following injection of histamine solutions from a multidose container[50] and postoperative, vein stripping, cutaneous infection traced to contaminated disinfectant.[205] The most frequent mycobacterial nosocomial pathogens so far reported belong to the so-called rapid-grower group. Undoubtedly, the nosocomial problem posed by these organisms is greater than is generally appreciated. This is due in part to a low level of suspicion and the failure of these organisms to be detected by routine bacterial culture methods. Unless specific acid-fast cultures are requested, these organisms (particularly the slower growers) consistently will be overlooked.

Mycoplasmatales

The fastidious microorganisms with no cell walls that are members of this family are obtained commonly from the oral cavity, upper respiratory tract, and genitourinary tract—presumably as normal flora. *Mycoplasma pneumoniae* is the major pathogen of the family, causing atypical pneumonia, but is rarely a significant nosocomial pathogen. However, immunosuppressed patients seem to develop more severe clinical syndromes when they are infected by *M pneumoniae*.[204] *Ureaplasma ureolyticum*, a common inhabitant of the genitourinary tract, and *M hominis*, which inhabits both the genitourinary tract and the upper respiratory tract, are of controversial significance. They have been implicated as causes of nongonococcal urethritis, but the supporting evidence is not overwhelming. Nosocomial blood invasion appears to be well documented, is usually transient, and tends to occur following vaginal deliveries,[390] cesarean section deliveries,[616] and therapeutic abortions[615] in women, and in urinary tract obstruction or manipulation in men.[562] There appears to be a correlation between these occurrences and tissue stresses at the sites of *Mycoplasma* carriage in the genitourinary tract. The relatively high neonatal colonization rate is also accounted for by this genitourinary tract carriage,[203, 332] although neonatal infections appear to be uncommon. Cultures from postoperative wound infections have yielded *M hominis* as a sole organism,[352] but such instances must be rare indeed. The need for special media and techniques to culture the Mycoplasmatales has limited the growth of our understanding of the role these microbes play in human disease.

Neisseria gonorrhoeae (gonococcus)

This gram-negative, oxidase-positive diplococcus is the cause of the most prevalent bacterial venereal disease. Its role in causing nosocomial infections is essentially limited to neonatal infection, whereby infants acquire the infection from their mothers. Such infections may be acquired in utero, during passage through the birth canal, or postpartum by direct contact with infected persons. The most notable infection of newborns by *N gonorrhoeae* is ophthalmia neonatorum. It has been standard procedure for years to instill silver nitrate into the eyes of neonates—a well-documented effective prophylactic measure. Despite this, however, occasional cases of infection still occur and are presumably due to either prenatal or postnatal infection—which would not be affected by silver nitrate instillation at birth.[608] In addition to ophthalmia, neonatal gonococcal infections (as determined by orogastric isolation of *N gonorrhoeae*) are associated with increased rates of prematurity, prolonged rupture of membranes, maternal peripartum fever, chorioamnionitis, and fetal death.[262]

Neisseria meningitidis (meningococcus)

This gram-negative, oxidase-positive diplococcus is a common normal inhabitant of the nasopharynx. The carriage rate is much higher ($>80\%$) during epidemics than during periods when there are no outbreaks. *N meningitidis* is among the three most common causes of bacterial meningitis, although nosocomial meningococcal meningitis is rare indeed. In fact, despite the fear in persons who attend such patients, the risk of acquisition of such infection is extremely low, and transmission requires extensive contact.[23] Prophylactic antimicrobics are recommended by many authorities for persons who come in close contact with meningitis patients. If the isolated *N meningitidis* is susceptible to sulfonamide, this would be the preferred drug. The increasing frequency of sulfonamide-resistant *N meningitidis* has led many to recommend minocycline or rifampin for such prophylaxis.

At least two forms of nosocomial meningococcal infections have been described, but to date they are relatively uncommon. (1) Neonatal meningococcal meningitis has been documented in infants born of mothers who have cervicovaginal colonization of *N meningitidis*, and presumably such infections are acquired during delivery.[101, 303] (2) Meningococcal pneumonia is being described with increasing frequency, and group Y appears to have a particular predilection for the respiratory tract. Nosocomial pneumonias due to *N meningitidis* do occur, and one outbreak in a cancer center was recently reported in which airborne transmission was suspected but not proved.[111] Since *N meningitidis* and other *Neisseria* species are common components of the upper respiratory airway, much caution must be exercised in the interpretation of *N meningitidis* isolated from sputum. Tracheal aspirate specimens would be more appropriate if meningococcal pneumonia is a real possibility.

Nocardia species

These species are aerobic, gram-positive, often partially acid-fast, branching bacilli. Nocardiae are generally considered environmental microbes and not normally part of the human flora. However, transient colonization by nocardiae is postulated as a source of human infection, particularly nosocomial infections in which an exogenous source is rarely, if ever, identified. Immunosuppressed patients, especially those receiving immunosuppressant therapy, have increased susceptibility to nosocomial nocardial infection.[30, 235, 337, 474, 669] *N asteroides* is the species most often associated with such infections, but other species such as *N caviae* are occasionally encountered.[474] Because Nocardiae are more slow-growing than most bacteria, they are not cultured by routine methods unless culture plates are held for at least four to seven days. They are grown quite readily, however, by standard mycobacterial and fungal culture methods.

Peptococcus and Peptostreptococcus species

These gram-positive, anaerobic cocci are normal components of the intestinal tract of humans and may be cultured with variable frequencies from the oral cavity, hair follicles of the skin, and genitourinary tract. These microbes are commonly isolated from nosocomial infections, particularly from postoperative wound infections.[477] They are usually found mixed with other organisms such as *S aureus* and *B fragilis*, and their possible synergistic role in such infections is postulated. However, in as many as 10% of such infections, the anaerobic cocci are isolated in pure culture, and thus their pathogenic potential is well documented.[477] Underlying debilitation is a common predisposing factor in these patients. Infections are virtually always of endogenous origin, and cross-infection is not a significant risk.

Phycomycetes

This group, also known as Zygomycetes, includes the genera *Mucor*, *Rhizopus*, and *Absidia*, among others. They are fungi with nonseptate hyphae. Phycomycetes are common in the environment and are cultured more often as laboratory contaminants than as significant clinical isolates. The Phycomycetes are nonpathogenic for persons with normal defense mechanisms. Infections occur, therefore, only in compromised patients and hence are often nosocomial. These infections are serious and often fatal. Certain underlying conditions appear to render patients particularly susceptible to phycomycoses. Patients with leukemia and lymphoma are much more susceptible than patients with solid cancers.[398, 458] Diabetes mellitus and corticosteroid therapy also appear to increase susceptibility.[398] Phycomycotic infections of burns are being seen with increasing frequency despite an overall decrease in burn infections. This is attributed to the use of topical antimicrobial agents such as mafenide (Sulfamylon), which has successfully suppressed bacterial infections such as those due to *P aeruginosa* but has allowed increased colonization of burns by fungi such as *Aspergillus* species and the Phycomycetes.[200, 429] Such fungal infections have a propensity to invade blood vessels with subsequent thrombosis and necrosis of adjacent tissue, which may require radical surgical intervention.[200]

The sources of Phycomycetes infections are considered to be exogenous, although the actual site is rarely documented. We have observed one case of nosocomial phycomycosis in which the cause was identified, although the actual mechanism was never proved. This was a case of palatal and maxillary sinus phycomycosis due to *Rhizopus oryzae* in an alcoholic with advanced cirrhosis, whose infection became manifest two days after a facial plastic surgical procedure. The surgery occurred in a new operating room (less than one month of use), and grain beetles were seen to emerge from the walls of the room during the day of this patient's surgery. Several beetles were ground up and cultured, as were portions of the plaster wall—both of which grew out the identical organism found in the patient. Limited air sampling yielded no growth of fungi. It appears probable that the source of this patient's infection was the operating room, and although airborne transmission is most likely, it was not demonstrated.

Recent outbreaks of *Rhizopus* species infections have been traced to contaminated elastic dressings.[109, 112, 222] The infections have been directly related to the use of these dressings, and they include postoperative wound infections, intravenous catheter site infections, buttocks abscesses in leukemic patients following iliac crest biopsies subsequently covered with elastic dressings to prevent bleeding, and a gastrointestinal infection in a premature infant in whom the same incriminated material was used to secure a nasogastric tube and an umbilical catheter.

Plasmodium species

These protozoan blood parasites cause malaria. Since the infection is transmitted normally by the *Anopheles* mosquito, one might be surprised to learn that nosocomial malaria does occur—though rarely. There are two recognized mechanisms of nosocomial malaria. (1) In posttransfusion malaria, plasmodia are transfused from an infected (presumably asymptomatic) donor to a recipient.[123, 149, 547] The plasmodial parasites can survive in refrigerated blood (3–5 C) for two to three weeks.[149] Platelet concentrate transfusion has also been reported as a source of malaria.[220] (2) Recrudescent malaria has been reported in patients who have been subjected to certain stressful stimuli such as an intravenous cholangiogram.[134]

Pneumocystis carinii

A protozoan tissue parasite, this organism characteristically infects the lungs, although other organs have been involved on rare occasions. The epidemiology and life cycles of *P carinii* have yet to be elucidated adequately. Current evidence suggests that the asymptomatic carrier is a significant reservoir and link in transmission of the organism. Healthy persons rarely, if ever, become clinically ill with *P carinii* infection, but subclinical experience with the organism does occur, since serologic studies show significant antibody levels in some healthy persons. Clinical infections occur primarily in two forms: (1) A so-called plasma cell pneumonitis of infancy, and (2) an interstitial pneumonitis (with few or no plasma cells) in immunosuppressed patients of all ages. In a review of 194 cases, over 64% occurred in patients with leukemia or lymphoma, 92% were white and the age-related attack rate was greatest in infants under one year of age, followed by children one to nine years of age.[634] In a series of 41 renal transplant patients dying with pneumonia, 10 (24%) were due to *P carinii*, and in this group the only factor that showed any significant predisposing correlation with *P carinii* infection was the duration of high-dose corticosteroid therapy ($\geq$40 mg/day) of prednisone.[506] Two cancer institutions have observed recent significant increases in the incidences of *P carinii* infection—in what were considered outbreak proportions.[472, 565] In one instance, based on epidemiologic studies, it was suggested—but not proved—that person-to-person communicability was a significant factor in the outbreak.[565] In another case, the outbreak was correlated with more intense immunosuppressive chemotherapy, with activation of latent *P carinii* infection postulated as the mechanism.[472] Although both these mechanisms remain plausible, neither has been proved. Communicability of such infections probably is relatively low, and except possibly in cancer units, isolation of such patients has shown no demonstrable benefit.

Propionibacterium acnes

An anaerobic gram-positive diphtheroid bacillus, this organism is a significant component of the normal cutaneous flora, residing primarily in hair follicles. Its prevalence in this site renders it a nuisance as a contaminant of specimens that are obtained via the percutaneous route, eg, blood cultures; but because infections by *P acnes* (eg, endocarditis) may rarely occur, such isolates cannot be dismissed automatically as skin contaminants. From a nosocomial infection standpoint, implements or tubings placed in percutaneous or subcutaneous positions for long periods of time are particularly susceptible to *P acnes* colonization and infection. The classic example is the ventriculoatrial shunt used in the treatment of patients with hydrocephalus, in which true *P acnes* infections are well documented.[52] *P acnes,* as well as other members of the genus, may be cultured from the flora of other sites such as fecal flora, and also may be obtained from polymicrobial wound infections, in which its pathogenic role is considered to be minimal.

Proteus mirabilis

This gram-negative bacillus belongs to the family Enterobacteriaceae. *P mirabilis* is a common inhabitant of the human intestinal tract and frequently colonizes other sites (eg, the upper respiratory tract and genital tract), particularly in hospital settings. It is a major nosocomial pathogen as judged by the frequency with which it is isolated from nosocomial infections at our institution; the majority of nosocomial *P mirabilis* infections are urinary tract infections, ranking third as a cause of nosocomial UTIs in our institution (see Table 3-1). It is presumed, and some evidence supports the concept, that the source of these infections is the fecal flora. Identical serotypes are often found in the urine and feces.[143] *P mirabilis* is also isolated with significant frequency from postoperative wound infections and respiratory infections (see Tables 4-1 and 5-1). Although bacteremias have been reported in as many as a third of nosocomial *P mirabilis* infections,[4] they occurred in only 2% of such infections in our experience (see Table 7-1). The majority of endemic nosocomial *P mirabilis* infections are of endogenous origin, but outbreaks of such infections are generally traceable to some exogenous source—either environmental contamination with *P mirabilis* (eg, humidifiers or suction devices)[51] or disseminating human carriers.[85] Neonates appear to be particularly susceptible to unusual *P mirabilis* infections and outbreaks, such as meningitis,[85, 561] osteomyelitis,[85, 360, 434] respiratory tract infections,[51] and sepsis.[85]

Because of the high prevalence of *P mirabilis* as a cause of nosocomial infection, some reliable form of typing or strain identification is highly desirable. A unique means of ascertaining the identity or nonidentity of two or more strains of swarming *Proteus* species is the Dienes test.[145] This determination is accomplished by observing the absence or presence of demarcation lines between two or more swarming strains inoculated simultaneously on an agar plate. The Dienes types seem to correlate best with proticine (*Proteus* bacteriocin) types.[567] The Dienes test does not always give reproducible results when used in a random fashion,[143, 276] but it appears to have considerable value in conjunction with other typing systems. Other typing systems for *P mirabilis* that have been valuable in epidemiologic studies include serotyping,[143, 567] protocine typing,[11, 315, 550] resistotyping,[315] and phage typing.[206, 276, 315, 540] We have found biotyping to be of limited value because of relatively poor reproducibility, at least in our hands. Because of the relative uniformity of antibiotograms among strains of *P mirabilis*, this technique has value only in identifying strains that show a significantly deviant pattern.

Providencia and indole-positive Proteus species

These members of the family Enterobacteriaceae are epidemiologically similar enough to be treated as a group. Specifically included herein are *Proteus vulgaris*, *Proteus morgani* (*Morganella morgani*), *Proteus rettgeri* (*Providencia rettgeri*), *Providencia stuartii*, and *Providencia alcalifaciens*. These species may be found in normal fecal flora but usually in relatively small numbers. The endemic nosocomial infection rate of these species is quite low, and even small clusters of such infections seriously raise the question of an outbreak. As with *P mirabilis*, most cause UTIs.[166, 575, 640, 653] Whereas endemic infections are usually of endogenous origin, epidemic infections are exogenous—either due to environmental contamination or via personnel.[166, 613, 640] In contrast with *P mirabilis* infections, however, these causative agents tend to be much more resistant to most antimicrobics,[166, 290, 451] infections tend to occur in patients who are receiving antimicrobics,[4, 166, 290] and infection rates increase with duration of hospitalization[4, 290] as well as with the presence and duration of indwelling urinary catheters.[290] Neurology patients, particularly paraplegics, seem particularly susceptible to *P rettgeri* infections.[290, 575] Burn infections caused by *P stuartii* have been reported with increasing frequency.[325, 451]

In most institutions the need to type such isolates rarely arises. Since the endemic level of these infections is so low, the presence of two or three infections by the same species usually will involve the same strain. If further strain identification is desired, biotyping of *P rettgeri* is often sufficient. Biotype 5 of *P rettgeri* has been shown to be merely a plasmid-mediated urease-positive *Providencia stuartii*.[180, 467, 469, 640] The Dienes test may be useful for determining the identity or nonidentity of two or more strains of *P vulgaris*, a swarming proteus. Serotyping appears to be the most practical of the typing methods currently available,[468, 575, 653] although antisera may not be readily available. Phage typing, bacteriocin typing, and resistograms typing have been described.[591]

Pseudomonas aeruginosa

This is a gram-negative, oxidase-positive, oxidative, nonfermentative bacillus. The organism is prevalent in the environment (eg, soil, food, water, and vegetables),[247, 556, 558, 602] which is the ultimate source of human colonization and infections. Ingestion of foods or liquids contaminated by *P aeruginosa* is followed by transient fecal colonization for usually less than one week,[82] but this can be prolonged by simultaneous administration of an antibiotic such as ampicillin. Identical strains of *P aeruginosa* have been isolated from hospital food and the subsequent fecal flora of patients who have ingested such food.[82, 556] That the carrier state is maintained by antimicrobic administration is supported by the finding of a higher fecal carriage rate in long-term hospital patients than in newly admitted patients.[560] Although such intestinal colonization is usually asymptomatic, especially in adults, it may produce intestinal infection with diarrhea of varying severity (even fatal) in neonates.[176] Outbreaks of neonatal *P aeruginosa* diarrhea have been traced both to human carriers[176] and to environmental sources such as contaminated breast milk pumps[606] and bathing detergents or receptacles.[130] The major significance of *P aeruginosa* colonization from an epidemiologic standpoint is that it provides a convenient source for endogenous nosocomial infections. In one study of 51 patients with nosocomial *P aeruginosa* infections, 37 (73%) were carriers, and 24 of these (65%) were infected with the same strains that they carried.[78]

P aeruginosa is not a primary pathogen, in the sense that it rarely produces infections in healthy individuals. Although immunocompromised patients generally show increased susceptibility to *P aeruginosa* infection, there are several specific conditions associated with the characteristic patterns of *P aeruginosa* infection. These include those listed below.

Cystic Fibrosis Patients.[339, 668]—The respiratory tracts of approximately half of such patients are colonized with *P aeruginosa*, which often is followed by pneumonia. The colonizing strains exhibit a characteristic mucoid quality that is rarely seen in any other condition. Although the mucoid variants tend to be more resistant to antimicrobics than the nonmucoid variants[238] and many cystic fibrosis patients receive antibiotics, this is not sufficient alone to explain the association of mucoid variants with cystic fibrosis. *P aeruginosa* infection of the lower respiratory tract is not an uncommon cause of death in these patients.

Burn Patients.[334, 363, 668]—Burn patients are unusually liable to become colonized and infected by *P aeruginosa*; the risk directly parallels the severity of the burn. In the past, such infections often resulted in sepsis with severe morbidity and not infrequently were the immediate cause of death. This is less of a problem now with the prevalent use of topical antimicrobial agents such as silver nitrate and mafenide (Sulfamylon), which has resulted in a significant reduction in the number of *P aeruginosa* infections—although in very severe burns the beneficial effect has been less than dramatic. Most, but not all, studies suggest that the environment is a more

important source of *P aeruginosa* burn infections than is intestinal colonization, and the hands of nurses and other patient attendants are the major
vectors.[26, 334, 363]

Neonates.[69, 159, 176, 194, 228, 416, 606]—Neonates are highly susceptible to *P
aeruginosa* enteric infections. Infection syndromes peculiar to neonates may
occur, such as noma neonatorum (gangrene of the lips and surrounding soft
tissue due to *P aeruginosa* infection, with sepsis and high mortality within
one to three days).[228] *P aeruginosa* infection outbreaks in newborn nurseries
are not rare and usually can be traced to environmental sources such as contaminated faucet aerators[194] and resuscitation equipment.[69, 159, 194] Neonatal
P aeruginosa infections tend to be more serious with a higher death rate
than comparable infections in adults.[416]

Malignancies.[196, 198, 471, 668]—A high proportion of nosocomial *P
aeruginosa* infections occur in patients who have malignant neoplastic
disease. Not only is there increased susceptibility in these patients, but also
there is a very substantial mortality from the infection. In these patients, the
severity of the infection and the risk of fatality correlate directly with (*a*)
severity of the underlying disease, (*b*) presence of bacteremia, (*c*) degree of
neutropenia, and (*d*) degree of hypogammaglobulinemia. In patients with
nosocomial infections, previous antibiotic therapy appears to be a significant preceding corollary. Unlike the other conditions described above, intestinal colonization appears to play a more important role in the epidemiology of infections in these patients than does environmental contamination.[539]

Miscellaneous.—The full spectrum of *P aeruginosa* nosocomial infections is virtually limitless. Besides the conditions mentioned above, other
features that are commonly associated with *P aeruginosa* infections include
broad-spectrum antibiotic therapy,[289, 668] inhalation therapy in cases of
respiratory infections,[289] and a traceable environmental source in cases of
nosocomial epidemics. The list of such environmental sources is also nearly
endless, but it includes such common items as sinks as a source of an ICU
outbreak,[602] faucet aerators as a source of postcardiac catheterization
wound infections,[135] Bigelow evacuators as a source of UTI outbreak,[415] ice
and ice-making machines as a source of an outbreak in a cardiothoracic
unit,[435] room humidifiers as a source of respiratory colonization and infection,[249] reused dialysis coils as a source of bacteremia outbreak,[621, 632] contaminated anesthesia machines as a source of respiratory tract colonization
and infection,[444] bar soaps, and germicide solutions.[78] Tracheostomy patients in ICUs are quite vulnerable to lower respiratory tract colonizations
and infection, and the contaminated hands of nursing personnel appear to
be the major immediate source of these microbes.[375] Of considerable
significance is the broad spectrum of antimicrobic resistance displayed by

P aeruginosa. But of even more concern is the emergence in the hospital environment of strains resistant to such drugs as carbenicillin and gentamicin, to which they are normally susceptible.[215, 374]

As suggested by the above list, *P aeruginosa* is a major nosocomial pathogen. The endemic level of nosocomial *P aeruginosa* infections varies considerably among institutions. In our hospital, *P aeruginosa* is the fifth most common isolate from all nosocomial infections, and more specifically ranks fifth for nosocomial postoperative wound infections (see Table 5-1), bacteremias (see Table 7-2), and respiratory tract infections (see Table 4-1), and fourth for UTIs (see Table 3-1).

Because of the widespread prevalence of *P aeruginosa*, it is important in epidemiologic investigations to be able to identify particular strains or to type these isolates. Several methods have been tried and found to be generally useful; these include pyocin typing (a form of bacteriocin typing),[177, 179, 239, 269, 373] phage typing,[59, 179] and serologic typing.[75, 414, 673] Mucoid variants are difficult to type by any system,[661, 673] but in cystic fibrosis patients the mucoid and nonmucoid variants in a particular patient are usually of the same type. Although opinions differ as to which one of the typing methods is most practical and useful, there is general agreement that the use of two or more systems in combination is more satisfactory.[58, 59, 60, 163, 341, 366] Endemic hospital strains of *P aeruginosa* tend to have quite characteristic antimicrobic susceptibility patterns, but when deviant patterns occur, these may serve as useful markers in following endemic and/or epidemic strains.[141] Once a problem appears to have been identified by common susceptibility patterns, it should be confirmed by a more conventional method.

Pseudomonas cepacia

This species is a gram-negative, motile, nonfermenting, aerobic bacillus. After *P aeruginosa*, *P cepacia* is the most significant nosocomial pathogenic member of the genus *Pseudomonas*. *P cepacia* is primarily an environmental organism, and human infections are virtually always exogenous in origin. This species is particularly resistant to cleaning and disinfectant solutions such as benzalkonium, cetrimide, and chlorhexidine, which thus may be contaminated by *P cepacia* and be an unsuspected source of infection. Most nosocomial *P cepacia* outbreaks can be traced to contaminated exogenous items. Examples include sepsis outbreaks traced to contaminated aqueous benzalkonium chloride used for skin decontamination,[208, 317] UTIs traced to contaminated detergicide (a quaternary ammonium compound) packaged in a commercial urinary catheter kit,[264] postoperative wound infections traced to contaminated Savlon (0.5% chlorhexidine and 0.5%

cetrimide) used for skin decontamination,[41] sepsis traced to contaminated pressure transducers,[103, 475] respiratory tract colonization and infection traced to contaminated local anesthetics used for bronchoscopy,[536] sepsis traced to contaminated multientry vials of saline used to mix medication,[89] and sepsis traced to contaminated serum albumin.[587] These examples illustrate the wide variety of infection and portals of entry that are quite characteristic for this organism.

Infections by *P cepacia* are more likely to occur and be severe in debilitated patients, and the majority of patients that become infected have been receiving antimicrobial chemotherapy.[162] *P cepacia* is normally the most antimicrobic-resistant member of the pseudomonads. It is not unusual for some isolates to be resistant to all drugs routinely tested. We recently encountered such an isolate causing an endocarditis of a prosthetic mitral valve. It was found to be susceptible only to an experimental antimicrobic (piperacillin) at 2 μg/ml. After one week of piperacillin therapy, the blood cultures became sterile. After two weeks, the valve was replaced, and the removed valve as well as postoperative blood cultures again grew out *P cepacia*—now resistant to piperacillin at greater than 512 μg/ml. The patient ultimately died of the infection. This antimicrobic resistance accentuates the need to prevent *P cepacia* infections, since the options for therapy are so limited.

Pseudomonas species

These are gram-negative, oxidase-positive, usually motile, aerobic bacilli with polar flagella. Members of the genus are ubiquitous in the environment and are usually associated with moisture. Although they are incriminated far less frequently than *P aeruginosa* as a cause of nosocomial infection, numerous species have been documented as occasional nosocomial pathogens. Examples include *P maltophilia*,[230, 231, 466, 549, 595] *P fluorescens*,[189, 231, 595] *P putrefaciens*,[625] *P stutzeri*,[231] and *P putida*.[466, 595] Even *P pseudomallei*, the cause of melioidosis, has been reported to produce recrudescent infections in a hospital setting—often following a surgical procedure.[515] The spectrum of nosocomial infections caused by these *Pseudomonas* species is as broad as those caused by *P aeruginosa* and includes UTIs, postoperative wound infections, abscesses, and sepsis. Different *Pseudomonas* species exhibit varying antibiotic susceptibility patterns, many of which are quite characteristic for a particular species and may be useful in confirming the identification as well as epidemiologic tracing.

Respiratory syncytial virus

This is a viral etiologic agent of a respiratory infection, primarily in children. Transmission is from person to person by air droplets or direct contact. Infections often occur in epidemics. Nosocomial outbreaks may occur synchronously with community-acquired epidemics; the source is usually a patient admitted to the hospital with a community-acquired infection. Personnel attending such a patient readily acquire the virus and serve as the major means of transmission to others. Risk of infection does not appear to be related to underlying disease or age, but it correlates best with length of stay in the unit in which the outbreak occurs.[260] Typically such nosocomial outbreaks occur in pediatric units or nurseries.[113, 118, 260] The frequency of such nosocomial infections is probably greater than generally appreciated due to the relative difficulty in accurately diagnosing the infection. Diagnosis is based on viral isolation or serologic studies, both of which are usually impractical in isolated infections but may be useful in outbreak situations.

Rhinovirus

This is the viral agent that most often causes the so-called common cold. The ubiquity and seasonal occurrence of this disease are familiar to all. Although little is written on the matter, it can be assumed that nosocomial rhinovirus infections occur with a frequency approaching that in the community. The significance of this has never been assessed to our knowledge, probably because of the relative benignancy of the infection. It is of interest to note that increasing evidence is accumulating that the hands are a significant means of rhinovirus transmission from person to person.[256] This again emphasizes the importance of appropriate hand-washing by hospital personnel.

Rhodotorula species

This reddish pigmented yeast is occasionally encountered as part of the upper respiratory tract flora and other flora in humans. Its pathogenic potential is low, but infections, including nosocomial infections, do occur rarely. In one report, there were two cases of nosocomial *Rhodotorula* fungemia secondary to prolonged intravenous cannulation, one of which resolved spontaneously upon removal of the cannula while the other required amphotericin B therapy.[353] Infections are usually rare and sporadic, and outbreaks have not been reported.

Rickettsia species

These organisms are bacteria-like obligate intracellular parasites. One of the characteristics of rickettsial infections (except Q fever) is that an arthropod vector is involved in the natural transmission of the microbe. Consequently, the potential for nosocomial infections by these microbes is quite limited. Patients with rickettsial infections may be rickettsiemic prior to clinical manifestation of the infection, and if they donate blood during this period, this blood may be the source of infection of the recipient. Such nosocomial infections have been documented for Rocky Mountain spotted fever and Q fever.[108, 647] Such infections, however, are rare and do not pose a major nosocomial infection problem.

Rotavirus

This viral agent has been implicated in diarrhea. Its epidemiology is still poorly understood. This is due in part to the difficulty with which it is detected—eg, via electron microscopy, which is not readily available to most laboratories. Nevertheless, diarrheal outbreaks in newborn and special care nurseries have been documented.[91, 125] The virus has been demonstrated in asymptomatic infants in these outbreaks, which raises the question of asymptomatic carriers. Underlying conditions do not appear to be significant predisposing factors. It is quite possible that this agent may be responsible for some of the nonbacterial diarrheas encountered in many nurseries, but until more practical methods of diagnosis are developed, this remains speculative.

Saccharomyces cerevisiae

This common large yeast has been recovered occasionally from clinical material, but it is generally not considered pathogenic. Rare cases have been reported in which true infection is suspected.[588] The prevalence of this organism may be greater than commonly appreciated, since in many laboratories it is not correctly identified. At the present time its importance in nosocomial infection appears quite minimal.

Salmonella enteritidis

This gram-negative enteric pathogen belongs to the family Enterobacteriaceae. Although asymptomatic carriers exist, this organism is not considered part of the normal flora. Most S enteritidis infections are community-acquired, but nosocomial outbreaks of salmonellosis are not rare. In the five-year period 1963–1967, 40 outbreaks of salmonellosis involving 3,025 patients and 43 deaths were reported to the CDC.[541] The actual prevalence is undoubtedly higher than this. Epidemiologically, two patterns of infection occur: (1) common source vehicle outbreaks, which are usually traced to food, most often eggs or egg products,[541, 586] and (2) person-to-person spread.[365, 541, 586] One report questions the importance of the latter mechanism. In this study, eight patients were admitted to the hospital with salmonellosis and with no enteric precautions for up to 72 hours, but the cultures taken from 265 exposed personnel and patients were negative.[378] However, this may be a reflection of good routine techniques rather than of the potential for person-to-person spread. Unusual means of transmission have also been implicated, such as a contaminated endoscope[122] and infected breast milk.[100] Common source food outbreaks tend to involve adults; these outbreaks are usually larger, less severe clinically, and easier to solve. Person-to-person outbreaks, often traced to asymptomatic carriers, tend to involve pediatric patients, are usually more severe clinically with a higher death rate, involve fewer patients, and are more difficult to solve.[541] More than 1,000 serotypes of *S enteritidis* are recognized based on somatic and flagellar antigens. Demonstration of a common serotype is an essential step in the investigation of a salmonellosis outbreak. Although such nosocomial outbreaks are relatively uncommon, it is important that they be detected early, be quickly and thoroughly investigated, and be ended as soon as possible.

Salmonella typhi and Salmonella choleraesuis

S typhi, a serious human pathogen, and *S choleraesuis* are rare causes of nosocomial infection today. When such infections occur, they usually are due to bizarre circumstances. For example, seven patients developed *S choleraesuis* sepsis following platelet transfusions during a six-month period. This was traced to a common donor found to have *S choleraesuis* osteomyelitis with asymptomatic bacteremia.[503]

Sarcoptes scabiei

This mite is the cause of scabies. Infestation by this mite is largely a nuisance and usually not clinically serious. Scabies is usually transmitted from person to person by direct contact. Although scabies is primarily a community-acquired infestation, nosocomial outbreaks may occur, particularly when undiagnosed patients are admitted to the hospital.[65]

Serratia species

These gram-negative, facultative, fermentative bacilli belong to the family Enterobacteriaceae. This genus is not a common component of normal flora in humans, although it is encountered occasionally. Until recently it was considered innocuous, but it is now recognized as a significant pathogen—primarily a nosocomial pathogen since the majority of its infections occur in the hospital setting. *S marcescens* is the major pathogenic species, accounting for more than 95% of the infections caused by members of the genus. We have encountered only one infection in five years due to *S rubidaea*. *S liquiefaciens* is seen slightly more often and has been reported by others as an occasional nosocomial pathogen.[639] *S marcescens* accounted for only 1.3% of nosocomial infections from 1975 to 1977 in our institution, but this is sharply less than the number five to ten years earlier, when several outbreaks of UTIs and RTIs occurred. Nosocomial outbreaks are characteristic of *S marcescens*. Such outbreaks are often traceable to a common source that is contaminated. Until its significance was realized and more adequate methods of decontamination and care were instituted, respiratory therapy equipment, especially nebulizers and humidifiers, were a major source of RTI outbreaks.[88, 178, 510, 531, 652] Contamination of solutions that are normally expected to be sterile has been the source of many outbreaks, eg, multientry medication bottles,[531] disinfectants,[178] plasma,[178] blood,[67] transducer fluids,[178] and irrigation fluids.[178] Person-to-person transmission by passive hand carriage by the nursing staff has been implicated in some outbreaks, particularly UTI outbreaks.[178, 383, 534] Although UTIs and RTIs are the most common manifestations of *S marcescens* infection, its spectrum is almost limitless, including wound infections,[655] intravenous catheter infections,[136, 153, 655] endocarditis,[490] and peritonitis.[136, 655] Septicemia is a common accompaniment of serious *S marcescens* infections.[136, 153, 655] Epidemiologic factors that seem to predispose to such infections include respiratory therapy,[136, 153, 178, 397] steroid therapy,[136, 153, 397] tracheostomies,[153] antimicrobic therapy,[136, 153, 397, 655] debilitating underlying disease,[136, 397, 655] recent surgical procedures,[136, 153, 397] and diabetes mellitus.[136] Steroid therapy and the presence of a tracheostomy often lead to a poor outcome from such infections.[153] In the investigation of *S marcescens* infections, both biotyping and serotyping are useful in strain identification, particularly when used in combination.[525] However, when the endemic infection rate is low, a sudden increase in *S marcescens* infections rarely requires sophisticated typing procedures in order to be recognized as a problem.

Shigella species

These gram-negative, nonmotile, facultative, fermentative bacilli belong to the family Enterobacteriaceae. Like *Salmonella* species, *Shigella* species are primary enteric pathogens and are not considered part of the normal intestinal flora of humans, although occasional asymptomatic long-term carriers are encountered.[358] Nosocomial *Shigella* species infections are not common and are more likely to occur in outbreaks in institutions with chronic long-term patients who have diminished ability for self-care, such as mental hospitals and nursing homes. Outbreaks may be spread by food[96, 154] or person to person.[97]

Staphylococcus aureus

These are gram-positive, catalase-positive, coagulase-positive cocci. *S aureus* is the prototype nosocomial pathogen of the antibiotic era, manifested by the prevalence and broad spectrum of infections it produces as well as its ability to develop resistance to antibiotics at a rate almost directly proportional to their usage. For the first two decades following the introduction of antibiotics, *S aureus* was by far the most important and frequent cause of nosocomial infections and outbreaks. Although it was superseded by gram-negative bacilli in the 1960s, it still remains a significant nosocomial pathogen. Countless studies, reports, reviews, and chapters have been published on the epidemiology of staphylococci, and no attempt to summarize these is possible here. However, a few pertinent comments are in order.

At any given time about a third of the general population harbors *S aureus* as part of their nasal or cutaneous flora; they are often referred to as carriers. Although there may be some racial differences in carrier rates (eg, blacks less than whites), no significant, consistent differences have been found associated with age, sex, or season.[408] Certain select populations, however, have been shown to have a significantly higher carrier rate—eg, insulin-requiring diabetics[569, 614] and chronic hemodialysis patients.[331]

The significance of the carrier state is twofold. First, *S aureus* carriers are more apt to develop staphylococcal infections than noncarriers—as exemplified by the increased incidence of *S aureus* infections among diabetics[569] and hemodialysis patients.[331] Second, carriers serve as an exogenous reservoir and source for *S aureus* infections in other patients.[27, 184, 265, 424] There is a very small subgroup of carriers who shed large numbers of organisms into their environments—commonly referred to as "shedders" or "disseminators,"[168, 265, 277] and they pose a more significant risk as a potential source of exogenous *S aureus* infections. This phenomenon may result, at least in infants (so-called cloud babies), from simultaneous infection by respiratory tract viruses.[168] Men are shedders more often than women.[277] Carriers fall into three general categories based on the duration and frequency of their carrier state: (1) persistent carriers—those who are consistently culture-positive for *S aureus*, usually of the same phage type, over long periods of time; (2) intermittent carriers—those whose carrier status alternates with periods of absence of *S aureus*; and (3) transient carriers—those who usually have negative cultures for *S aureus*, but who infrequently may become colonized for a short period of time. *S aureus* is not an indigenous environmental organism, and it will survive for only a relatively short time (a few days) in an inanimate environment. The source of *S aureus* infections is rarely primarily environmental, although fomites may serve as transient vectors of transmission. The source is either the person's own flora (endogenous) or the flora of another person (exogenous), which may be transmitted by direct contact, airborne dissemination, or contaminated fomites—in decreasing order of importance. The clothing of carriers is also a potential source.[577] Nosocomial outbreaks of S aureus infections are always exogenous infections, but the mechanism of spread may vary.

Since there is a close correlation between the colonization rate and the incidence of S aureus infections, efforts have been directed toward reducing the colonization rates in patients and personnel. These attempts often have resulted in the anticipated reductions in infection rates. This relationship has been dramatically exemplified during the past few years in newborn nurseries, where S aureus infections present serious problems. For years, the S aureus colonization and infection rate had been at an acceptably low level, largely due to the use of hexachlorophene bathing of newborn infants on a routine basis. With the demonstration of cutaneous absorption of hexachlorophene by neonates, particularly premature infants, and the potential CNS damage that can result from high systemic levels of this compound, the practice of routine hexachlorophene bathing of neonates was discontinued in most nurseries. This was followed by an abrupt increase in S aureus epidemics in newborn nurseries throughout the country. This inverse relationship between hexachlorophene bathing and S aureus colonization and infections is well documented.[202, 288, 362, 426, 439] This is not to say that hexachlorophene is the only means available for reducing S aureus colonization in nurseries, for it is not—nor is it without other undesirable side effects. For example, studies have shown that concomitant with the reduction of S aureus colonization is an increase in colonization by P aeruginosa and other gram-negative bacteria,[202, 362, 439] which are also significant potential pathogens for the newborn. This inverse relationship between the colonization of S aureus and that of gram-negative bacilli is not unique to neonates. For example, laminar flow isolation and prophylactic antimicrobics have been used successfully to reduce the number of gram-negative gut flora and infections in leukemia patients, but this treatment is often accompanied by a simultaneous increase in the colonization and infection rate by S aureus.[478]

Factors related to the pathogenesis of S aureus are not fully understood, but they include both bacterial factors such as toxins (eg, exfoliative toxin, usually produced by strains of phage group II or occasionally group I, which produces the so-called scalded skin syndrome)[174] and host factors such as breaks in normal protective barriers and debilitating underlying diseases such as diabetes, malignancies, and chronic renal and hepatic diseases.[127, 420, 438] Although any part of the body may be the site of an S aureus infection, soft tissue and bone are the most common sites today.[420] Despite its frequency as a community-acquired infection, S aureus osteomyelitis is only occasionally nosocomial.[422] Most nosocomial S aureus infections are soft-tissue infections, such as postoperative wound infections and abscesses.[559] S aureus pneumonia, an extremely serious infection, which was a relatively common nosocomial infection one to two decades ago, is seldom seen today. Nosocomial S aureus bacteremia and sepsis are common and serious complications of infection at specific sites and have an associated mortality as high as 42%.[127] The most common primary sites (many are not identified) are postoperative wound infections and infected intravascular devices.

As mentioned above, S aureus has the capacity to develop resistance to many antimicrobics. In most hospitals today, more than 90% of nosocomial S aureus infections are resistant to penicillin, ie, are β-lactamase producers. With the availability of β-lactamase-resistant penicillins (methicillin, nafcillin, oxacillin), the frequency and seriousness of noso-comial S aureus infections have diminished—although it is unclear what role these drugs played in the decrease. Although methicillin-resistant S aureus infection outbreaks have been reported,[332, 450] and the frequency of such infections may be rising,[55] they still do not present a major problem in most institutions in the United States. Gentamicin-resistant S aureus infec-tions and outbreaks are also being encountered but do not present a generalized problem at this time.[579, 629] It is of considerable interest that both gentamicin-resistant and methicillin-resistant S aureus strains appear to have a limited capacity to colonize in persons who are not receiving systemic antibiotics.[450, 579]

Because of the prevalence of S aureus as a colonizing and infecting agent, it is important to be able to type or subspeciate this organism when an outbreak is suspected. Although biotyping is the simplest method for do-ing this, the limited variation in biochemical reactions and the relatively poor reproducibility of many reactions render biotyping of limited usefulness. The standard and classical method is phage typing.[68] This, however, is not a simple procedure, and currently probably less than half a dozen US laboratories offer this test. Phage typing can be obtained through state laboratories at the CDC when outbreaks due to S aureus are suspected epidemiologically. Resistotyping has been suggested as a useful method of S aureus typing—particularly in combination with phage typing,[170] and perhaps this should be considered for non-phage-typable strains.

Our experience during the past few years suggests that S aureus out-breaks are much less common today than they were a decade or more ago. In the past five years we observed three clusters of S aureus infections (two in newborn nurseries) that were considered possible outbreaks, but in each instance phage typing at the CDC demonstrated multiple strains in each cluster, indicating no common source problem. Most nosocomial *S aureus* infections today are probably endogenous, although many are due to hospital *S aureus* that colonize the patient shortly after admission. *S aureus* remains a major nosocomial pathogen. In our hospital it is second only to *E coli* in frequency as a cause of all nosocomial infections and is the leading isolate from postoperative wound infections (see Table 5-1) and nosocomial bacteremias (see Table 7-2).

Staphylococcus epidermidis

This is a gram-positive, catalase-positive, coagulase-negative coccus. *S epidermidis* is a significant component of the normal flora of the skin, nose, oropharynx, urethra, and vagina. Long considered a nonpathogen, it is now recognized as a significant pathogen in sites associated with implanted foreign devices such as prosthetic heart valves[120, 578] and ventriculoatrial shunts.[495, 590] When it is isolated as the sole organism from an infection at a site that is normally sterile, it is usually accepted as a pathogen—eg, post-cataract-extraction endophthalmitis.[623] When isolated from sources in which it is frequently found as a contaminant, its role as a pathogen is far more controversial—a good example is urinary tract infections. Nevertheless, considerable evidence has been presented in recent years that strongly supports the role of *S epidermidis* as a cause of UTIs, not only cystitis but even acute pyelonephritis.[32, 462, 658] Utilizing the previously described criteria for nosocomial urinary tract infections, *S epidermidis* accounted for 7.4% of such infections in our hospital from 1975 to 1977 (see Table 3-1), ranking fifth in frequency.

S epidermidis infections are almost always of endogenous origin, and outbreaks caused by this species are rare. Since outbreaks are not observed, phage typing has little practical value,[598] but biotyping is occasionally of considerable value. This is particularly true for evaluating the significance of *S epidermidis* isolated from more than one blood culture from a patient.[57] Since the skin is heavily colonized by *S epidermidis*, blood cultures procured via venipuncture are occasionally contaminated by this organism. However, the cutaneous *S epidermidis* usually are represented by multiple biotypes. Hence, if multiple blood cultures grow *S epidermidis* of more than one type, contamination is likely; conversely, if only one biotype is represented, a true bacteremia must be strongly considered. By this standard, 7.4% of nosocomial bacteremias in our hospital were due to *S epidermidis* (see Table 7-2), ranking sixth in this category. *S epidermidis* readily lends itself to biotyping.[33, 34, 57] Some of the biotypes of *S epidermidis* are sufficiently distinct that they may eventually merit separate species status—in fact, *S saprophyticus* epidemiologically differs from other biotypes by being less frequently a component of the cutaneous flora, and it characteristically produces UTIs in young women. It does not appear to be a significant nosocomial organism at this time.

Streptococcus pyogenes

This group A streptococcus is gram-positive and catalase-negative and reacts to Lancefield group A antisera. This is the cause of the classic strep throat. By means of its toxins, it also is responsible for scarlet fever and erysipelas. Its infections may be followed by serious sequelae such as rheumatic fever and acute glomerulonephritis. The organism is not an environmental microbe, and humans are the primary reservoir and source of *S pyogenes* infections. Although *S pyogenes* is not considered part of the normal pharyngeal flora, asymptomatic "carriers" of *S pyogenes* do exist and presumably are important reservoirs for the organism between infections and outbreaks. Most *S pyogenes* infections today are community-acquired, and compared with the pre-antibiotic era, nosocomial *S pyogenes* infections are relatively uncommon. *S pyogenes* accounts for less than 1% of nosocomial infections in our institution but was isolated from 1.3% of postoperative wound infections from 1975 to 1977 (see Table 5-1). Wound infections are generally the most common type of nosocomial *S pyogenes* infections; they are usually sporadic and the sources are rarely determined. However, outbreaks do occur even today and usually can be traced to someone among the hospital personnel who is an asymptomatic carrier. Usually those are pharyngeal carriers, but some recent outbreaks have been traced to asymptomatic anal carriers and vaginal carriers.[253, 393, 535, 584] This illustrates the extent to which it is necessary to go to track down the sources of some outbreaks. Such personnel carriers should not be permitted to continue working in sensitive areas such as operating rooms until their carrier status has been treated and eradicated. Puerperal sepsis, a major nosocomial *S pyogenes* infection problem in the past, has been almost eliminated since the beginning of the antibiotic era, but rare outbreaks may still occur.[298] *S pyogenes* bacteremias are relatively uncommon in patients who have the usual community-acquired pharyngitis, but they are more apt to occur in patients who have the types of infections that are nosocomial. In two studies of *S pyogenes* bacteremias, more than half were nosocomial.[258, 271] In both, postoperative wound infections were the most common identified source, followed by lower respiratory tract infections and a scattering of miscellaneous infections.

In suspected outbreaks, the presence of a single etiologic strain or type can be confirmed by serologic subtyping using the M, T, or R antigen system. This technique is not available in most routine clinical laboratories but can be performed easily by state or other reference laboratories.

Streptococcus agalactiae

This group B streptococcus is gram-positive and catalase-negative and reacts with Lancefield group B antisera. In the past decade, this organism has emerged as a significant nosocomial pathogen. This is due in part to the availability of simpler methods for its identification by routine clinical laboratories, and in part to a true increase in the prevalence of *S agalactiae* infections in recent years. The epidemiology of this organism is not well understood. It is generally stated that the female and male genitourinary tracts are the major reservoir for *S agalactiae*. Based on better selective culture methods, it would appear that about a fourth of women are vaginal carriers. However, studies comparing genitourinary tract carriage with fecal carriage have shown that all vaginal carriers are fecal carriers, and the fecal carrier rate is higher than the vaginal—suggesting that the fecal reservoir may be primary and the source of genitourinary colonization.[31, 411, 460] As with staphylococci, the carrier status for *S agalactiae* may be persistent, intermittent, or transient.[22, 192]

Pharyngeal colonization by *S agalactiae* occurs at a rate of 10%–15% and is not significantly different in patients with pharyngitis and in normal controls.[191] The colonization sites and frequency are of significance because of the nature of the infection to which they give rise. Neonatal *S agalactiae* infection is the most common serious group B streptococcal infection seen today, and *S agalactiae* has become the most common cause of neonatal sepsis and meningitis.[36] Nearly 50% of infants born of vaginally colonized mothers become colonized on passage through the birth canal—common sites of colonization are the ear canals and umbilicus.[192] The neonatal infection rate, however, is considerably lower. Prolonged rupture of membranes appears to increase the risk of neonatal infection.[350] An important factor in the risk of neonatal infection (besides colonization of the birth canal) is the presence or absence of maternal antibodies to *S agalactiae* (with placental transfer to the infant). It appears that such antibodies protect the infant, and neonatal infections occur almost exclusively in infants without such protection.[37, 38]

Two forms of neonatal infection are recognized clinically. (1) Early-onset infection usually becomes manifest within five days after birth—often within the first few hours. This type appears to be clearly of maternal origin and is fulminant with extremely high mortality. Clinically and radiographically, it may closely resemble hyaline membrane disease.[2, 270, 321] The infection is one of overwhelming sepsis with major pulmonary involvement, but meningitis is less prevalent in this form than in the late-onset form. Early diagnosis is usually missed because of the frequent absence of the usual signs and symptoms of infection. It should be suspected in low-birth-weight infants who have unexplained apneic episodes during the first few hours of life.[491] There is usually no increased amount of IgM. (2) Late-onset infection usually becomes manifest after ten days of life. Although sepsis may occur, meningitis is the most frequent manifestation. When the infection is appropriately treated, the mortality is significantly less than that of the early-onset infection. The source of S agalactiae in late-onset disease is not always clear, but potential sources include endogenous infection from colonization after passage through the birth canal, intimate contact with maternal carrier, contact with hospital staff carrier, and passive transmission by personnel from another colonized or infected infant. Reduction in the infant colonization rate has been reported after the use of triple-dye (brilliant green, proflavine, and crystal violet) treatment of the umbilicus.[633]

Group B streptococcal nosocomial infections are not limited to infants. Postpartum endometritis and sepsis[45, 356] and even meningitis[252, 356] in women are not rare. Other adult infections, all of which may be accompanied by septicemia, include pneumonia,[45] urinary tract infections including pyelonephritis,[45, 356] meningitis, postoperative wound infections,[356] and burn "infections" with autograft rejection.[573] In adults, S agalactiae acts opportunistically, infecting patients with underlying conditions such as malignancies, diabetes mellitus, steroid therapy, and chronic liver and renal diseases.[356] In our experience from 1975 to 1977, S agalactiae was cultured from 2.5% of postoperative wound infections (see Table 5-1) and 1.5% of nosocomial UTIs (see Table 3-1); it accounted for 1.5% of all nosocomial bacterial and fungal infections.

Currently five serotypes of S agalactiae are recognized. Attempts to correlate serotypes with specific infections have resulted in conflicting reports. However, several patterns are emerging. Type III accounts for the overwhelming majority of S agalactiae neonatal meningitis[35, 656, 657] and early-onset septicemia,[21, 35] but less than half of the cases of late-onset sepsis.[35] These data suggest an increased infectious potential for type III in neonates, particularly meningeal infection. Adult infections show a more even distribution of serotypes.[270, 356] There is a definite potential for outbreaks due to S agalactiae, especially in newborn nurseries, and serotyping may be of some value in establishing these.

Streptococcus group D

These gram-positive, catalase-negative cocci react with Lancefield group D antisera. This group of organisms is conveniently subdivided into two subgroups by various biochemical tests such as salt tolerance. The enterococci (tolerant to 6.5% sodium chloride) are particularly resistant to multiple antimicrobial agents, whereas nonenterococci (salt-intolerant) tend to be much more susceptible to antibiotics. Both enterococci and nonenterococci are normal inhabitants of the intestinal tract. In abnormal bowel conditions such as ulcerative colitis, however, the prevalence of group D streptococci may be increased a hundredfold.[626] Enterococci are more prevalent and far more common causes of nosocomial infections, and the most common species among the enterococci is *S faecalis*, which accounts for more than 90% of nosocomial enterococcal infections. The most frequent *S faecalis* nosocomial infections are UTIs, and this species was the second most frequent cause of such infections in our institution, accounting for 9.0% of nosocomial UTIs between 1975 and 1977 (see Table 3–1). In one interesting report, *S faecalis* was the most common cause of UTIs in renal transplant patients and was associated with subsequent graft rejection.[87] The second most frequent nosocomial site from which *S faecalis* is isolated is postoperative wound infections (see Table 5–1). Its role in such infections is somewhat uncertain because it is almost never isolated in pure culture from wounds but is usually mixed with other potential pathogens such as gram-negative bacilli, anaerobes, and staphylococci. However, *S faecalis* septicemia occasionally does occur with such infections, indicating that in at least some cases it plays a pathogenic role.[161, 182] It is of some interest that the *liquefaciens* variety of *S faecalis* was isolated from wounds twice as often as the non-*liquefaciens* variant (see Table 5–1). Whether this has any significance remains to be determined.

Nosocomial group D streptococcal infections are almost always of endogenous origin, and consequently nosocomial outbreaks rarely, if ever, occur with this group. Although serotyping of this group can be done, it appears to have little practical epidemiologic value at this time.

Streptococcus pneumoniae

Also called *Pneumococcus* or *Diplococcus pneumoniae*, this gram-positive, catalase-negative diplococcus does not react to Lancefield grouping sera. The reservoir for this organism is the upper respiratory tract of humans, and approximately 5% of normal asymptomatic persons carry the organism.[158] There appears to be some seasonal variation in the carrier rate, being somewhat higher in the winter months than in the summer, and this correlates with the seasonal variation in the prevalence of pneumococcal pneumonia in some populations.[329] *S pneumoniae* is the leading cause of community-acquired bacterial pneumonia, but it is a lesser threat as a nosocomial pathogen. Nevertheless, nosocomial pneumococcal pneumonias do occur. By using the NNIS criteria for nosocomial respiratory tract infections, 6.3% of nosocomial respiratory infections in our hospital from 1975 to 1977 were due to *S pneumoniae* (see Table 4–1). Bacteremia frequently accompanies such infections. *S pneumoniae* is a recognized cause of infection at many other sites, such as meningitis and peritonitis, which are seldom nosocomial.

A number of underlying conditions increase the risk of patients acquiring pneumococcal infections and dying of these infections. Hospitalized patients with malignancies, especially leukemia, lymphoma, and myeloma, who are also receiving immunosuppressive chemotherapy and/or corticosteroids are at increased risk, with greater than 50% mortality.[201] In recent years, much attention has been devoted to the increased risk of patients who have had a splenectomy. This risk is greatest in infants and young children during the first two years after surgery, and in patients with underlying reticuloendothelial malignancies.[66] Even otherwise healthy individuals who have undergone splenectomy are subject to a slightly increased risk of infection, but more important, such infections are often fulminant with a high death rate.[236] Patients with hyposplenism due to medical diseases (eg, sickle cell anemia) have similar risks.[66, 546] These patients appear to be appropriate candidates for polyvalent pneumococcal polysaccharide vaccines, which recently have become available and have been shown to both elicit appropriate antibody responses in such patients and be protective.[19, 568] Serotyping of pneumococci is available and may be useful epidemiologically.

Streptococcus, non-groups A, B, D, and nonpneumococcus

These gram-positive, catalase-negative cocci do not react to groups A, B, D, or pneumococcal antisera. Although most streptococcal infections are caused by the previously described species, occasional infections, both community-acquired and nosocomial, are caused by less common species.[161, 182, 451, 483] These include species belonging to Lancefield groups C and E through T as well as nontypable species. Of these, those most often reported as causes of nosocomial infections are group C,[73, 161, 182] group F,[39, 73, 161, 182] group G,[161, 182, 278] group H,[182] group K,[73, 182] group L,[182] group M,[76] and nongroupable species.[161, 182] Most of these are cultured from wound infections and abscesses. Since most of those implicated groups are normal components of the pharyngeal flora, as well as those of the skin, vagina, and occasionally the intestinal tract, it is likely that most infections by them are endogenous. Outbreaks have been reported but are distinctly uncommon.[278]

Streptomyces species

These gram-positive, conidia-forming filamentous microbes are environmental organisms normally found in the soil. Infections caused by them are virtually limited to mycetomas. Otherwise this species is considered to be nonpathogenic and, when isolated from other clinical sources, is considered to be a contaminant. There is, however, at least one documented case of neonatal pneumonia due to *S pellitieri*.[649] Since the same organism was isolated from the mother's vagina, it is probable that the infection was acquired during the infant's passage through the birth canal. How the mother became colonized is not known. Although it is highly unlikely that such an infection will be encountered in US hospitals, it is mentioned here to reemphasize the point that microbes normally considered contaminants must be given more serious consideration when they are isolated from compromised hosts.

Strongyloides stercoralis

This is a small intestinal nematode. Strongyloidiasis, often considered a tropical disease, is endemic in many parts of the United States, particularly the southern and southeastern states. The free-living form is found in moist soil. The infective or filariform larvae penetrate the skin of humans, usually the feet, and are passively carried by the bloodstream to the lungs. They penetrate the ventilatory system and migrate to the pharynx, where they are swallowed and settle in the small intestine. Here they mature, and the adult female lays eggs that usually hatch before defecation. The resulting rhabditiform larvae are usually passed in the feces, and normal further development occurs in the soil. Autoinfections may occur, or if filariform larvae develop in the intestinal tract, they may reenter the bloodstream via the gut mucosa or perianal skin. The severity of symptoms generally is proportional to the numbers of organisms in the lungs and intestine. However, infestations may persist in a relatively latent and asymptomatic phase for years. When such patients are subjected to immunosuppressive insults, the infection may become systemic, with the involvement of many organs, including the brain. Such "hyperinfections" have occurred in patients who have lymphoreticular malignancies[509, 514, 544] and in patients who are receiving immunosuppressive therapy, especially corticosteroids, for a variety of diseases.[137, 175, 432, 509, 544] These overwhelming infections are often fatal, largely because the diagnosis is not suspected clinically. It is recommended that patients who are to receive such immunosuppressive therapy and are from endemic areas of the country or world should be checked for the presence of these parasites before therapy and treated if present. Person-to-person spread of strongyloidiasis is not a significant means of transmission, and nosocomial hyperinfections appear to be reactivations of latent infections.

Torulopsis glabrata

This small, budding yeast is found as part of the normal pharyngeal, vaginal, and intestinal flora of many humans. It usually is considered a nonpathogen but is being seen with increasing frequency as an opportunistic pathogen. The typical setting is a patient with major underlying disease who is receiving antimicrobic and immunosuppressive chemotherapy.[7, 384, 454, 622] The spectrum of infections is broad in this setting. *T glabrata* fungemia may be secondary to infections of other sites but also is often associated with colonized intravenous catheters, particularly hyperalimentation lines.[259, 384, 622] In the latter instances the fungemia is often transient and will resolve upon removal of the intravenous line. Likewise, *T glabrata* may be cultured from the urine of catheterized patients in counts greater than 10^5/ml, but these fungurias usually remit spontaneously upon removal of the catheter.[384] However, true urinary tract infections—even renal infections—may occur, particularly in diabetic patients.[322] Pneumonias due to *T glabrata* have been reported in patients who are severely myelosuppressed from either their underlying disease or chemotherapy.[8] In our 1975-1977 experience, *T glabrata* was isolated from 1.4% of the nosocomial UTIs (see Table 3-1) and 1.1% of nosocomial respiratory infections (see Table 4-1). A period of asymptomatic colonization appears to precede the appearance of infections at most sites.[7] In nearly all series studied, including our own, antibiotic therapy is a factor—either concurrent with or immediately preceding the onset of *T glabrata* infections. Infections appear to be endogenous, and nosocomial outbreaks have not been reported.

Toxoplasma gondii

This is a unicellular parasite whose life cycle is incompletely understood. It is considered primarily an animal parasite, and the usual means of transmission to humans is ingestion of raw or inadequately cooked, infected meat. Oocysts are commonly present in cat feces, and there is some evidence to suggest that the infection rate is higher in people who have close contact with cats, although conflicting reports also exist. The typical infection in adults is a mononucleosis-like syndrome with fever and lymphadenopathy—a benign self-limited disease. A third means of transmission is transplacental from mother to infant. This is a much more severe form of infection, with cerebral and retinal involvement.

None of these usual means of acquiring toxoplasmosis is nosocomial, but nosocomial infections do occur, and two additional mechanisms of transmission have been implicated. First, a few reports have implicated the transplantation of an infected organ or transfusion of infected leukocytes.[502, 524] Such instances are rare, and this mode of transmission has not been proved. The second mechanism is a result of a defect in cellular immunity that permits the recrudescence of a latent infection.[527] This is supported by the fact that the majority of such cases occur in patients who have serious underlying diseases such as malignancies,[1, 93, 128, 232, 524, 527, 605, 627, 654] collagen-vascular disease,[232, 527] and renal homografts[128, 232, 502, 527] and who are receiving corticosteroids or other immunosuppressive therapy. In these cases the illness is usually disseminated and has a predilection for central nervous system involvement; this illness is fatal if untreated. In most instances, unfortunately, the infection is not suspected and the patient dies before a diagnosis is made. Of epidemiologic importance is the observation that there is a high prevalence of concomitant DNA viral infections—herpes simplex and cytomegalovirus infections.[232, 527, 627] Because of the nature of acquisition, nosocomial outbreaks do not occur.

Trichosporon species

This is a yeast-like fungus that produces hyphae and arthrospores. Members of this genus are occasionally cultured from the normal flora of humans from various sites. Its pathogenicity is largely limited to the skin and hair—eg, white piedra. However, there are rare case reports of systemic infection in debilitated patients. Examples include infective endocarditis of a prosthetic mitral valve and renal infection and sepsis in a renal transplant patient—both due to *T cutanecum*,[379] and disseminated infection including endocarditis in a bone marrow transplant patient due to *T capitatum*.[665] Such infections are undeniably rare but point out the severity of iatrogenic immunosuppression.

Vaccinia virus

This attenuated pox virus is used to vaccinate against smallpox. Patients with leukemia or lymphoma, particularly when they are receiving corticosteroids and/or other immunosuppressive agents, are particularly susceptible to systemic vaccinial infections when vaccinated for smallpox.[433, 455, 520, 619] Such infections, often referred to as progressive vaccinia or vaccinia necrosum, are often fatal if untreated. With the virtual elimination of smallpox from the globe, there is now little reason for such infections to occur. The use of vaccinia vaccination in the treatment of herpetic ulcers and other cutaneous viral infections has been shown to have no value.

Varicella zoster virus

This DNA virus of the herpesvirus group causes both varicella (chicken-pox) and herpes zoster. With this virus, the host–parasite relationship is complex and incompletely understood. The usual primary infection, varicella, is a common, relatively benign and self-limited childhood illness, which is highly contagious and normally transmitted via upper respiratory tract secretions—prior to the cutaneous eruptions. Following the active disease, the virus becomes a dormant or latent resident of sensory nerve ganglia, and in the majority of individuals it remains indefinitely. If, however, the person's immune status, especially cellular immunity, becomes impaired by either some disease process or iatrogenic therapy, the virus may become reactivated and may produce the entity herpes zoster, which may be local along the sensory distribution of one or two nerves or, less commonly, disseminated. The disseminated variety is extremely serious and often fatal.

From a nosocomial epidemiologic standpoint, several aspects must be considered. Since varicella is a relatively benign disease and highly con-tagious, children who have it should not be admitted to the hospital. If they must be admitted, they should be placed in strict isolation and cared for by people with known immunity to the virus. Unfortunately, the period of communicability begins several days prior to the clinical illness, and if such patients are admitted to a pediatric ward during this prodrome period without a diagnosis, nosocomial outbreaks are likely to occur.[99] Since many pediatric hospitalized patients are already very ill, the acquisition of varicella can be devastating—particularly in leukemic patients and those who are receiving corticosteroids. In such patients the infection may pro-duce pneumonia, encephalitis, and ultimately death.[99, 326]

Zoster seems to show a clear predilection for patients who have malignancies[186, 233, 388, 538, 663] and those receiving immunosuppressive therapy.[492, 497] Among the malignancies, lymphoma patients are more susceptible to zoster than those with other cancers;[186, 538] but among the lymphomas, Hodgkin's disease is by far the leader in the incidence of com-plicating zoster, varying from 15% to 35% in different series.[186, 233, 499, 538, 663] Additional factors that increase the risk even more in patients with Hodgkin's disease are advanced stage of the disease, immunosuppressive chemotherapy, extensive radiation therapy, cutaneous anergy, and possibly splenectomy, but reports are conflicting on the latter. From 15% to 27% of such cases represent disseminated zoster, which is a far more serious prob-lem, and there is some increased association between the disseminated form and intensive chemotherapy.[233] The effect of zoster infection on patients with Hodgkin's disease is also unclear. In one series, no adverse effect in terms of relapse of Hodgkin's disease or fatality was noted,[499] yet another report showed that when zoster occurred more than six months after therapy for Hodgkin's disease, it heralded a relapse in 10 of 13 cases.[663] In any event, patients with zoster are infectious and should be placed in isolation and nursed by personnel who are immune to varicella. Since zoster and varicella are actually host manifestations of infection by the same virus, either or both manifestations may occur in the same outbreak. Demonstration of varicella acquired from zoster patients is quite firm, but the converse is not so clearly proved.[61] Furthermore, the distinction between disseminated varicella and disseminated zoster is a moot one.

Veillonella species

These gram-negative anaerobic cocci occur as part of the normal upper respiratory tract and intestinal flora of humans. They are occasionally isolated from nosocomial infections, most often wound infections, and almost invariably are mixed with other potential pathogens. Their role in such infections currently is not clear.

Yersinia enterocolitica

This gram-negative facultative bacillus belongs to the family Enterobacteriaceae. It is not considered normal in human flora and, like *Salmonella* species, it is an enteric pathogen. It is also a common cause of mesenteric lymphadenitis—producing an appendicitis-like syndrome clinically. In outbreaks, the pathogens are usually foodborne. However, a recently reported nosocomial outbreak appears to have occurred via person-to-person spread.[611] We have encountered one postoperative wound infection from which this organism was isolated, and it is probable that the full infection spectrum of *Y enterocolitica* (and *Y pseudotuberculosis*) has not been elucidated yet. This is due in part to the fact that practical methods for isolating and recognizing the bacillus in fecal cultures are not generally available. When the organism is isolated from other sites, it is often not adequately differentiated from other Enterobacteriaceae.

REFERENCES

1. Abell C, Holland P: Acute toxoplasmosis complicating leukemia. Diagnosis by bone marrow aspiration. Am J Dis Child 118:782–787, 1969

2. Ablow RC, et al: A comparison of early onset group B streptococcal neonatal infections and the respiratory-distress syndrome of the newborn. N Engl J Med 294:65–70, 1976

3. Abrams E, Zierdt CH, Brown JA: Observations on *Aeromonas hydrophila* septicemia in a patient with leukemia. J Clin Pathol 24:491–492, 1971

4. Adler JL, Burke JP, Martin DF, Finland M: *Proteus* infections in a general hospital. II. Some clinical and epidemiological characteristics with an analysis of 71 cases of *Proteus* bacteremia. Ann Intern Med 75:531–536, 1971

5. Ahmad FJ, Darrell JH: Significance of the isolation of *Clostridium welchii* from routine blood culture. J Clin Pathol 29:185–186, 1976

6. Airo R, Apollonio T, Pranzo A: Neonatal meningitis due to *Mima polymorpha*. Lancet 2:611–612, 1971

7. Aisner J, et al: *Torulopsis glabrata* infection in patients with cancer. Increasing incidence and relationship to colonization. Am J Med 61:23–28, 1976

8. Aisner J, et al: *Torulopsis glabrata* pneumonitis in patients with cancer. Report of three cases. JAMA 230:584–585, 1974

9. Akhtar M, Young I: Measles giant cell pneumonia in an adult following long-term chemotherapy. Arch Pathol 96:145–148, 1973

10. Albritton WL, Wiggins GL, Feeley JC: Neonatal listerosis: distribution of serotypes in relation to age at onset of disease. J Pediatr 88:481–483, 1976

11. Al-Julaili IS: Bacteriocine typing of *Proteus*. J Clin Pathol 28:784–787, 1975

12. Alpern RJ, Dowell VR Jr: *Clostridium septicum* infection and malignancy. JAMA 209:385–388, 1969

13. Alpern RJ, Dowell VR Jr: Nonhistotoxic clostridial bacteremia. Am J Clin Pathol 55:717–725, 1971

14. Alter HJ, et al: Health-care workers positive for hepatitis B surface antigen. Are their contacts at risk? N Engl J Med 292:454–457, 1975

15. Alter HJ, et al: Posttransfusion hepatitis after exclusion of commercial and hepatitis-B antigen-positive donors. Ann Intern Med 77:691–699, 1972

16. Alter HJ, et al: Type B hepatitis: The infectivity of blood positive for e antigen and DNA polymerase after accidental needlestick exposure. N Engl J Med 295: 909–913, 1976

17. Altmann G, Horowitz A, Kaplinsky N, Frankl O: Prosthetic valve endocarditis due to *Mycobacterium chelonei*. J Clin Microbiol 1:531–533, 1975

18. Altmann G, Sechter I, Cahan D, Gerichter CB: *Citrobacter diversus* isolated from clinical material. J Clin Microbiol 3:390–392, 1976

19. Ammann AJ, et al: Polyvalent pneumococcal-polysaccharide immunization of patients wtih sickle-cell anemia and patients wtih splenectomy. N Engl J Med 297:897–900, 1977

20. Anderson GS, Penfold JB: An outbreak of diphtheria in a hospital for the mentally subnormal. J Clin Pathol 26:606–615, 1973

21. Anthony BF, Concepcion NF: Group B *Streptococcus* in a general hospital. J Infec Dis 132:561–567, 1975

22. Anthony BF, Okada DM, Hobel CJ: Epidemiology of group B *Streptococcus*: longitudinal observations during pregnancy. J Infect Dis 137:524–530, 1978

23. Artenstein MS, Ellis RE: The risk of exposure to a patient with meningococcal meningitis. Milit Med 133:474–477, 1968

24. Ashcraft KW, Leape LL: *Candida* sepsis complicating parenteral feeding. JAMA 212:454–456, 1970

25. Atherton ST, White DJ: Stomach as source of bacteria colonising respiratory tract during artificial respiration. Lancet 2:968–969, 1978

26. Atuk NO, Hunt EH: Serial tuberculin testing and isoniazid therapy in general hospital employees. JAMA 218:1795–1798, 1971

27. Ayliffe GAJ, Collins BJ: Wound infection acquired from a disperser of an unusual strain of *Staphylococcus aureus*. J Clin Pathol 21:195–198, 1967

28. Ayliffe GAF, Lowbury EJL: Sources of gas gangrene in hospitals. Br Med J 2:333–336, 1969

29. Ayliffe GAJ, et al: *Pseudomonas aeruginosa* in hospital sinks. Lancet 2:578–581, 1974

30. Bach MC, et al: Influence of rejection therapy on fungal and nocardial infections in renal-transplant recipients. Lancet 1:180–184, 1973

30. Bach MC, et al: Influence of rejection therapy on fungal and nocardial infections in renal-transplant recipients. Lancet 1:180–184, 1973

31. Badri MS, et al: Rectal colonization with group B *Streptococcus*: relation to vaginal colonization of pregnant women. J Infect Dis 135:308–312, 1977

32. Bailey RR: Significance of coagulase-negative *Staphylococcus* in urine. J Infect Dis 127:179–182, 1973

33. Baird-Parker AC: A classification of micrococci and staphylococci based on physiological and biochemical tests. J Gen Microbiol 30:409–427, 1963

34. Baird-Parker AC: The classification of staphylococci and micrococci from world-wide sources. J Gen Microbiol 38:363–387, 1965

35. Baker CJ, Barrett FF: Group B streptococcal infections in infants. The importance of the various serotypes. JAMA 230:1158–1160, 1974

36. Baker CJ, et al: Suppurative meningitis due to streptococci of Lancefield group B: A study of 33 infants. J Pediatr 82:724–729, 1973

37. Baker CJ, Kasper DL: Correlation of maternal antibody deficiency with susceptibility to neonatal group B streptococcal infection. N Engl J Med 294:753–756, 1976

38. Baker CJ, Kasper DL: Immunologic investigation of infants with septicemia or meningitis due to group B *Streptococcus*. J Infec Dis 136(supp):S98–S104, 1977

39. Bannantyne RM, Randall C: Ecology of 350 isolates of group F *Streptococcus*. Am J Clin Pathol 67:184–186, 1977

40. Bartlett JG, Chang TW, Gurwith M, Gorbach SL, Onderdonk AB: Antibiotic-associated pseudomembranous colitis due to toxin-producing clostridia. N Engl J Med 298:531–534, 1978

41. Bassett DCJ, Stokes KJ, Thomas WRG: Wound infection with *Pseudomonas multivorans*. A water-borne contaminant of disinfectant solutions. Lancet 1:1188–1191, 1970

42. Bassett HFM, et al: Sources of staphylococcal infection in surgical wound sepsis. J Hyg 61:83, 1963

43. Bast RC Jr, Zbar B, Borsos T, Rapp HJ: BCG and cancer. N Engl J Med 290:1413–1420, 1458–1469, 1974

44. Bayer AS, Blumenkrantz MJ, Montgomerie JZ, Galpin JE, Coburn JW, Guze LB: *Candida* peritonitis: report of 22 cases and review of the English literature. Am J Med 61:832–840, 1976

45. Bayer AS, Chow AW, Anthony BF, Guze LB: Serious infections in adults due to group B streptococci. Clinical and serotypic characterization. Am J Med 61:498-503, 1976

46. Bayer AS, Chow AW, Betts D, Guze LB: Lactobacillemia—report of nine cases. Important clinical and therapeutic considerations. Am J Med 64:808-813, 1978

47. Bayer AS, Edwards JE Jr, Seidel JS, Guze LB: *Candida* meningitis: report of seven cases and review of the English literature. Medicine 55:477-486, 1976

48. Bayer AS, Nelson SC, Galpin JE, Chow AW, Guze LB: Necrotizing pneumonia and empyema due to *Clostridium perfringens*: Report of a case and review of the literature. Am J Med 59:851-856, 1975

49. Beck A, O'Brien PK, Mackenzie VF: Case of stillbirth due to infection with *Listeria monocytogenes*. J Clin Pathol 19:567-569, 1966

50. Beck A, Stanford JL, Inman PM, Brown AE: Mycobacteria, skins, and needles. Lancet 2:801, 1969

51. Becker AH: Infection due to *Proteus mirabilis* in newborn nursery. Am J Dis Child 104:355-359, 1962

52. Beeler BA, Crowder JG, Smith JW, White A: *Propionibacterium acnes*: Pathogen in central nervous system shunt infection. Report of three cases including immune complex glomerulonephritis. Am J Med 61:935-938, 1976

53. Beem MD, Saxon EM: Respiratory-tract colonization and a distinctive pneumonia syndrome in infants infected with *Chlamydia trachomatis*. N Engl J Med 296:306-310, 1977

54. Belsey MA, Sinclair M, Roder MA, LeBlanc DR: *Corynebacterium diphtheriae* skin infections in Alabama and Louisiana—a factor in the epidemiology of diphtheria. N Engl J Med 280:135-141, 1969

55. Benner EJ, Kayser FH: Growing clinical significance of methicillin-resistant *Staphylococcus aureus*. Lancet 2:741-744, 1968

56. Bennett JV: Human infections: economic implications and prevention. Ann Intern Med 89:761-763, 1978

57. Bentley DW, Haque R, Murphy RA, Lepper MN: Biotyping, an epidemiological tool for coagulase-negative staphylococci. Antimicrob Agents Chemother 1967:54-59, 1968

58. Bergan T: Epidemiological markers for *Pseudomonas aeruginosa*. 1. Serogrouping, pyocine typing—and their interrelationships. Acta Pathol Microbiol Scand B 81:70-80, 1973

60. Bergan T: Epidemiological markers for *Pseudomonas aeruginosa*. 3. Comparison of bacteriophage typing, serogrouping, and pyocine typing on a heterogeneous clinical material. Acta Pathol Microbiol Scand B 81:91–101, 1973

61. Berlin BS, Campbell T: Hospital-acquired herpes zoster following exposure to chickenpox. JAMA 211:1831–1833, 1970

62. Bettelkeim KA, Dulake C, Taylor J: Post-operative urinary infections caused by *Escherichia coli*. J Clin Pathol 24:442–443, 1971

63. Bernouilli C, et al: Danger of accidental person-to-person transmission of Creutzfeldt-Jakob disease. N Engl J Med 290:692–693, 1977

64. Bieger RC, Brewer NS, Washington JA II: *Haemophilus aphrophilus*: a microbiologic and clinical review and report of 42 cases. Medicine 57:345–355, 1978

65. Biro L, Price E: An "epidemic" of scabies. JAMA 226:1568, 1973

66. Bisno AL: Hyposplenism and overwhelming pneumococcal infection: a reappraisal. Am J Med Sci 262:101–107, 1971

67. Black WA, Pollock A, Batchelor EL: Fatal transfusion reactions due to *Serratia marcescens*. J Clin Pathol 20:883–886, 1967

68. Blair JE, Carr AB: The techniques and interpretation of phage typing of staphylococci. J Lab Clin Med 55:650–661, 1960

69. Bobo RA, et al: Nursery outbreaks of *Pseudomonas aeruginosa*: Epidemiological conclusions from five different typing methods. Appl Microbiol 25:414–420, 1973

70. Bockemühl J, Pan-Urai R, Burkhardt F: *Edwardsiella tarda* associated with human disease. Pathol Microbiol 37:393–401, 1971

71. Bodner SJ, Koenig MG, Goodman JS: Bacteremic *Bacteroides* infections. Ann Intern Med 73:537–544, 1970

72. Bojsen-Møller J: Human listerosis: Diagnostic, epidemiological and clinical studies. Acta Pathol Microbiol Scand B (suppl) 229:1–157, 1972

73. Braunstein H, Tucker E, Gibson BC: Infections caused by unusual beta hemolytic streptococci. Am J Clin Pathol 55:424–430, 1971

74. Britt MR: Infectious diseases in small hospitals; prevalence of infections and adequacy of microbiology services. Ann Intern Med 89:757–760, 1978

75. Brokopp, CD, Gomez-Lus R, Farmer JJ III: Serological typing of *Pseudomonas aeruginosa*: Use of commercial antisera and live antigen. J Clin Microbiol 5:640–649, 1977

76. Broome CV, Moellering RC Jr, Watson BK: Clinical significance of Lancefield groups L-T streptococci isolated from blood and cerebrospinal fluid. J Infect Dis 133:382–392, 1976

77. Brown C, Seidler RJ: Potential pathogens in the environment: *Klebsiella pneumoniae*, a taxonomic and ecological enigma. Appl Microbiol 25:900–904, 1973

78. Bruun JN, McGarrity GJ, Blakemore WS, Coriell LL: Epidemiology of *Pseudomonas aeruginosa* infections: determination of pyocine type. J Clin Microbiol 3:264–271, 1976

79. Bryan JA, Carr HE, Gregg MB: An outbreak of nonparenterally transmitted hepatitis B. JAMA 223:279–283, 1973

80. Buchholz DH, et al: Bacterial proliferation in platelet products stored at room temperature. Transfusion-induced *Enterobacter* sepsis. N Engl J Med 285:429–433, 1971

81. Buchman TG, Roizman B, Adams G, Stover BH: Restriction endonuclease fingerprinting of herpes simplex virus DNA: a novel epidemiologic tool applied to a nosocomial outbreak. J Infect Dis 138:488–498, 1978

82. Buck AC, Cooke EM: The fate of ingested *Pseudomonas aeruginosa* in normal persons. J Med Microbiol 2:521–525, 1969

83. Buffenmyer CL, Rycheck RR, Yee RB: Bacteriocin (klebocin) sensitivity typing of *Klebsiella*. J Clin Microbiol 4:239–244, 1976

84. Bulger RJ, Sherris JC: The clinical significance of *Aeromonas hydrophila*. Arch Intern Med 118:562–564, 1966

85. Burke JP, et al: *Proteus mirabilis* infections in a hospital nursery traced to a human carrier. N Engl J Med 284:115–121, 1971

86. Buxton AE, Anderson RL, Werdegar D, Atlas E: Nosocomial respiratory tract infection and colonization with *Acinetobacter calcoaceticus*. Epidemiologic characterization. Am J Med 65:507–513, 1978

87. Byrd LH, et al: Association between *Streptococcus faecalis* urinary infections and graft rejection in kidney transplantation. Lancet 2:1167–1169, 1978

88. Cabrera HA: An outbreak of *Serratia marcescens* and its control. Arch Intern Med 123:650–655, 1969

89. Cabrera HA, Drake MA: An epidemic in a coronary care unit caused by *Pseudomonas* species. Am J Clin Pathol 64:700–704, 1975

90. Cabrera A, Tsukada Y, Pickren JW: Clostridial gas gangrene and septicemia in malignant disease. Cancer 18:800–806, 1965

91. Cameron DJS, Bishop RF, Veenstra AA, Barnes GL: Noncultivable viruses and neonatal diarrhea: Fifteen-month survey in a newborn special care nursery. J Clin Microbiol 8:93–98, 1978

92. Capps RB, Sborov V, Scheiffley CS: A syringe-transmitted epidemic of infectious hepatitis. JAMA 136:819–824, 1948

93. Carey RM, Kimball AC, Armstrong D, Lieberman PH: Toxoplasmosis. Clinical experiences in a cancer hospital. Am J Med 54:30–38, 1973

94. Casewell M, Phillips I: Food as a source of *Klebsiella* species for colonization and infection of intensive care patients. J Clin Pathol 31:845–849, 1978

95. Caul EO, et al: Cytomegalovirus infections after open heart surgery. A prospective study. Lancet 1:777–781, 1971

96. Center for Disease Control: Shigellosis—North Carolina. Morbid Mortal Weekly Rep 18:11–16, 1969

97. Center for Disease Control: Shigellosis outbreak—Utah. Morbid Mortal Weekly Rep 18:123, 1969

98. Center for Disease Control: Follow-up on septicemias associated with contaminated Abbot intravenous fluids. Morbid Mortal Weekly Rep 20:91–92, 1971

99. Center for Disease Control: An outbreak of varicella on a pediatric ward. Morbid Mortal Weekly Rep 20:127–128, 1971

100. Center for Disease Control: *Salmonella kottbus* meningitis associated with contaminated breast milk. Morbid Mortal Weekly Rep 20:154, 1971

101. Center for Disease Control: Meningococcal meningitis in an infant. Morbid Mortal Weekly Rep 20:323–324, 1971

102. Center for Disease Control: Septicemias associated with contaminated intravenous fluids. Morbid Mortal Weekly Rep 22:99, 1973

103. Center for Disease Control: Nosocomial *Pseudomonas cepacia* bacteremia caused by contaminated pressure transducers. Morbid Mortal Weekly Rep 23:423, 1974

104. Center for Disease Control: False-positive blood cultures related to the use of evacuated nonsterile blood-collection tubes—Georgia, Massachusetts. Morbid Mortal Weekly Rep 24:387–388, 1975

105. Center for Disease Control: Primary bacteremia—Illinois. Morbid Mortal Weekly Rep 25:110/115, 1976

106. Center for Disease Control: Atypical mycobacterial wound infection. Morbid Mortal Weekly Rep 25:233–243, 1976

107. Center for Disease Control: Isolation of mycobacteria species from porcine heart valve prostheses. Morbid Mortal Weekly Rep 26:42–43, 1977

108. Center for Disease Control: Q fever—California. Morbid Mortal Weekly Rep 26:86–91, 1977

109. Center for Disease Control: Nosocomial outbreak of *Rhizopus* infections associated with Elastoplast wound dressings—Minnesota. Morbid Mortal Weekly Rep 27:33–34, 1978

110. Center for Disease Control: Follow-up on mycobacterial contamination of porcine heart valve prostheses. Morbid Mortal Weekly Rep 27:92/98, 1978

111. Center for Disease Control: Nosocomial transmission of Group Y *Neisseria meningitidis* in cancer patients. Morbid Mortal Weekly Rep 27:147–153, 1978

112. Center for Disease Control: Follow-up on *Rhizopus* infection associated with Elastoplast bandages—United States. Morbid Mortal Weekly Rep 27:243–244, 1978

113. Center for Disease Control: Nosocomial respiratory syncytial virus infection in an intensive care nursery—California. Morbid Mortal Weekly Rep 27:260–267, 1978

114. Center for Disease Control: Legionnaires' disease—Los Angeles, California. Morbid Mortal Weekly Rep 27:394–399, 1978

115. Center for Disease Control: National Nosocomial Infections Study Report, Annual Summary 1975. October 1977.

116. Center for Disease Control, Hospital Infections Section: Outline for surveillance and control of nosocomial infections. June 1977.

117. Chang RS, et al: Oropharyngeal excretion of Epstein-Barr virus by patients with lymphoproliferative disorders and recipients of renal homografts. Ann Intern Med 88:34–40, 1978

118. Chanock RM, et al: Respiratory syncytial virus. JAMA 176:647, 1961

119. Chatterjee SN, et al: Primary cytomegalovirus and opportunistic infections. JAMA 240:2446–2449, 1978

120. Cheng TO, Kinhal V, Tice DA: Fatal thrombosis of the Starr-Edwards mitral valve prosthesis associated with bacterial endocarditis. Chest 57:151–155, 1970

121. Chetlin SH, Elliott DW: Preoperative antibiotics in biliary surgery. Arch Surg 107:319–323, 1973

122. Chmel H, Armstrong D: *Salmonella oslo*. A focal outbreak in a hospital. Am J Med 60:203–208, 1976

123. Chojnacki RE, Brazinsky JH, Barrett D Jr: Transfusion—introduced falciparum malaria. N Engl J Med 279:984–985, 1968

124. Chow AW, Guze LB: *Bacteroidareae* bacteremia: clinical experience with 112 patients. Medicine 53:93–126, 1974

125. Chrystie IL, et al: Rotavirus infections in a maternity unit. Lancet 2:79, 1975

126. Clarke JS, et al: Preoperative oral antibiotics reduce septic complications of colon operations: results of prospective, randomized, double-blind clinical study. Ann Surg 186:251–259, 1977

127. Cluff LE, Reynolds RC, Page DL, Breckenridge JL: Staphylococcal bacteremia and altered host resistance. Ann Intern Med 69:859–873, 1968

128. Cohen SN: Toxoplasmosis in patients receiving immunosuppressive therapy. JAMA 211:657–660, 1970

129. Cooke EM, Hettiaratchy IGT, Buck AC: Fate of ingested *Escherichia coli* in normal persons. J Med Microbiol 5:361–369, 1972

130. Cooke EM, Shooter RA, O'Farrell SM, Martin DR: Fecal carriage of *Pseudomonas aeruginosa* by newborn babies. Lancet 2:1045–1046, 1970

131. Corey L, et al: HB_SAg-negative hepatitis in a hemodialysis unit: Relation to Epstein-Barr virus. N Engl J Med 293:1273–1277, 1975

132. Coyle-Gilchrist MM, Crewe P, Roberts G: *Flavobacterium meningosepticum* in the hospital environment. J Clin Pathol 29:824–826, 1976

133. Craig WA, et al: Hospital use of antimicrobial drugs, survey of 19 hospitals and results of antimicrobial control program. Ann Intern Med 89:793–795, 1978

134. Crosby DJ, Storm AH: Malarial relapse induced by intravenous cholangiography. Arch Intern Med 118:79–80, 1966

135. Cross DF, Benchimol A, Dimond EG: The faucet aerator—a source of *Pseudomonas* infection. N Engl J Med 274:1430–1431, 1966

136. Crowder JG, Gilkey GH, White AC: *Serratia marcescens* bacteremia. Clinical observations and studies of precipitin reactions. Arch Intern Med 128:247–253, 1971

137. Cruz T, Reboucas G, Rocha H: Fatal strongyloidiasis in patients receiving corticosteroids. N Engl J Med 275:1093–1096, 1966

138. Curtis JR, Wing AJ, Coleman JC: *Bacillus cereus* bacteremia, a complication of intermittent haemodialysis. Lancet 1:136–138, 1967

139. Davis TJ, Matsen JM: Prevalence and characteristics of *Klebsiella* species: relation to association with a hospital environment. J Infect Dis 130:402–405, 1974

140. Davis WA II, Kane JG, Garagusi VF: Human *Aeromonas* infections. Medicine 57:267–277, 1978

141. Dayton SL, Blasi D, Chipps DD, Smith RF: Epidemiological tracing of *Pseudomonas aeruginosa*; antibiogram and serotyping. Appl Microbiol 27:1167–1169, 1974

142. Deinhardt F: Epidemiology and mode of transmission of viral hepatitis A and B. Am J Clin Pathol 65:890–897, 1976

143. deLouvois J: Serotyping and the Dienes reaction on *Proteus mirabilis* from hospital infections. J Clin Pathol 22:263–268, 1969

144. De Vita VT, Utz JP, Williams T, Carbone PP: *Candida* meningitis. Arch Intern Med 117:527–535, 1966

145. Dienes L: Reproductive processes in *Proteus* cultures. Proc Soc Exp Biol Med 63:265–270, 1946

146. Dienstag JL, et al: Etiology of sporadic hepatitis B surface antigen-negative hepatitis. Ann Intern Med 87:1–6, 1977

147. Dienstag JL, et al: Fecal shedding of hepatitis A antigen. Lancet 1:765–767, 1975

148. Dienstag JL, Szmuness W, Stevens CE, Purcell RH: Hepatitis A virus infection: New insights from seroepidemiologic studies. J Infect Dis 137:328–340, 1978

149. Dike AE: Two cases of transfusion malaria. Lancet 2:72–73, 1972

150. Dismukes WE, Royal SA, Tynes BS: Disseminated histoplasmosis in corticosteroid-treated patients. JAMA 240:1495–1498, 1978

151. Dixon RE: Effect of infections on hospital care. Ann Intern Med 89:749–753, 1978

152. Dmochowski L: Viral type A and type B hepatitis. Morphology, biology, immunology and epidemiology—A review. Am J Clin Pathol 65:741–786, 1976

153. Dodson WH: *Serratia marcescens* septicemia. Arch Intern Med 121:145–150, 1968

154. Donadio JA, Gangarosa EJ: Foodborne shigellosis. J Infect Dis 119:666–668, 1969

155. Dorff GJ, Jackson LJ, Rytel MW: Infection with *Eikenella corrodens*. A newly recognized human pathogen. Ann Intern Med 80:305–309, 1974

156. Doshi R: *Aspergillus fumigatus* endocarditis of an aortic homograft with aneurysm of the ascending aorta. J Pathol 103:263–265, 1970

157. Douglas RG Jr, et al: Herpes simplex virus pneumonia: occurrence in an allotransplanted lung. JAMA 210:902–904, 1969

158. Dowling JN, Sheehe PR, Feldman HA: Pharyngeal pneumococcal acquisition in "normal" families: a longitudinal study. J Infect Dis 124:9–17, 1971

159. Drewett SE, Payne DJH, Tuke W, Verdon PE: Eradication of *Pseudomonas aeruginosa* infection from a special care nursery. Lancet 1:946–948, 1972

160. Duffy P, et al: Possible person-to-person transmission of Creutzfeldt-Jakob disease. N Engl J Med 290:692–693, 1974

161. Duma RJ, Weinberg AN, Medrek TF, Kunz LJ: Streptococcal infections. A bacteriological and clinical study of streptococcal bacteremia. Medicine 48:87–127, 1969

162. Ederer GM, Matsen JM: Colonization and infection with *Pseudomonas cepacia*. J Infect Dis 125:613–618, 1972

163. Edmonds P, Suskind RR, MacMillan BG, Holder IA: Epidemiology of *Pseudomonas aeruginosa* in a burn hospital: evaluation of serological, bacteriophage, and pyocin typing methods. Appl Microbiol 24:213–218, 1972

164. Edmondson EB, Sanford JP: The *Klebsiella-Enterobacter (Aerobacter) Serratia* group. Medicine 46:323–340, 1967

165. Edwards JE Jr, Foos RY, Montgomerie JZ, Guze LB: Ocular manifestations of *Candida* septicemia: review of seventy-six cases of hematogenous *Candida* endophthalmitis. Medicine 53:47–75, 1974

166. Edwards LD, Gross A, Levin S, Landau W: Outbreak of a nosocomial infection with a strain of *Proteus rettgeri* resistant to many an timicrobials. Am J Clin Pathol 61:41–46, 1974

167. Ehrenkranz NJ, Kicklighter JL: Tuberculosis outbreak in a general hospital: evidence for airborne spread of infection. Ann Intern Med 77:377–382, 1972

168. Eichenwald HF, Kotsevalov O, Fasso LA: The "cloud baby": an example of bacterial-viral interaction. Am J Dis Child 100:161–173, 1960

169. Elek SD, Higney L: Resistogram typing—a new epidemiological tool; application to *Escherichia coli*. J Med Microbiol 3:103–110, 1970

170. Elek SD, Moryson C: Resistotyping of *Staphylococcus aureus*. J Med Microbiol 7:237–249, 1974

171. Englund GW: Persistent septicemia due to *Hafnia alvei*. Report of a case. Am J Clin Pathol 51:717–719, 1969

172. Epstein MA, Achong BG: Various forms of Epstein-Barr virus infections in man: established fact and a general concept. Lancet 2:836–839, 1973

173. Eras P, Goldstein MJ, Sherlock P: *Candida* infection of the gastrointestinal tract. Medicine 51:367–379, 1972

174. Faden HS, Burke JP, Glasgow LA, Everett JR III: Nursery outbreak of scalded-skin syndrome. Scarlatiniform rash due to phage group I *Staphylococcus aureus*. Am J Dis Child 130:265–268, 1976

175. Fagundes LA, Busato O, Brentano L: Strongyloidiasis: fatal complication of renal transplantation. Lancet 2:439–440, 1971

176. Falcão DP, et al: Nursery outbreak of severe diarrhoea due to multiple strains of *Pseudomonas aeruginosa*. Lancet 2:38–40, 1972

177. Falkiner FR, Keane CT: Epidemiological information from active and passive pyocine typing of *Pseudomonas aeruginosa*. J Med Microbiol 10:447–459, 1977

178. Farmer JJ III, et al: Detection of *Serratia* outbreaks in hospital. Lancet 2:455–459, 1976

179. Farmer JJ III, Herman LG: Epidemiological fingerprinting of *Pseudomonas aeruginosa* by the production of and sensitivity to pyocin and bacteriophage. Appl Microbiol 18:760–765, 1969

180. Farmer JJ III, et al: Unusual Enterobacteriaceae: *"Proteus rettgeri"* that "change" into *Providencia stuartii*. J Clin Microbiol 6:373–378, 1977

181. Farrar WE: Serious infections due to "non-pathogenic" organisms of the genus *Bacillus*. Am J Med 34:134, 1963

182. Feingold DS, Stagg NL, Kunz LJ: Extrarespiratory streptococcal infections. Importance of the various serologic groups. N Engl J Med 275:356–361, 1966

183. Feinstone FM, et al: Transfusion-associated hepatitis not due to viral hepatitis type A or B. N Engl J Med 292:767–770, 1975

184. Fekety FR Jr: The epidemiology and prevention of staphylococcal infection. Medicine 43:593–613, 1964

185. Feld R, Bodey GP, Groschel D: Mycobacteriosis in patients with malignant disease. Arch Intern Med 136:67–70, 1976

186. Feldman S, Hughes WT, Kim HY: Herpes zoster in children with cancer. Am J Dis Child 126:178-184, 1973

187. Feldman WE: *Bacteroides fragilis* ventriculitis and meningitis. Am J Dis Child 130:880-883, 1976

188. Fellner JM, Dowell VR Jr: "Bacteroides" bacteremia. Am J Med 50:787-796, 1971

189. Felsby M, Munk-Andersen G, Siboni K: Simultaneous contamination of transfusion blood with *Enterobacter agglomerans* and *Pseudomonas fluorescens*, supposedly from the pilot tubes. J Med Microbiol 6:413-416, 1973

190. Felts SK, et al: Sepsis caused by contaminated intravenous fluids: epidemiologic, clinical, and laboratory investigations of an outbreak in one hospital. Ann Intern Med 77:881-890, 1972

191. Ferrieri P, Blair LL: Pharyngeal carriage of group B streptococci: detection by three methods. J Clin Microbiol 6:136-139, 1977

192. Ferrieri P, Cleary PP, Seeds AE: Epidemiology of group-B streptococcal carriage in pregnant women and newborn infants. J Med Microbiol 10:103-114, 1977

193. Fiala M, et al: Epidemiology of cytomegalovirus infection after transplantation and immunosuppression. J Infect Dis 132:421-433, 1975

194. Fierer J, Taylor PM, Gezon HM: *Pseudomonas aeruginosa* epidemic traced to delivery-room resuscitators. N Engl J Med 276:991-996, 1967

195. Finland M: Changing ecology of bacterial infections as related to antibacterial therapy. J Infect Dis 122:419-431, 1970

196. Fishman LS, Armstrong D: *Pseudomonas aeruginosa* bacteremia in patients with neoplastic disease. Cancer 30:764-773, 1972

197. Fishman LS, Griffin JR, Sapico FL, Hecht R: Hematogenous *Candida* endophthalmitis—a complication of candidemia. N Engl J Med 286:675-681, 1972

198. Flick MR, Cluff LE: Pseudomonas bacteremia. Review of 108 cases. Am J Med 60:501-508, 1976

199. Foley FD, et al: Herpesvirus infection in burned patients. N Engl J Med 282:652-656, 1970

200. Foley FD, Shuck JM: Burn-wound infection with Phycomycetes requiring amputation of hand. JAMA 203:596, 1968

201. Folland D, Armstrong D, Seides S, Blevins A: Pneumococcal bacteremia in patients with neoplastic disease. Cancer 33:845-849, 1974

202. Forfar JO, Gould JC, MacCabe AF: Effect of hexachlorophene on incidence of staphylococcal and gram-negative infection in the newborn. Lancet 2:177–180, 1968

203. Foy HM, Kenny GE, Levinsohn EM, Grayston JT: Acquisition of mycoplasmata and T-strains during infancy. J Infect Dis 121:579–587, 1970

204. Foy HM, et al: *Mycoplasma pneumoniae* infections in patients with immunodeficiency syndromes: report of four cases. J Infect Dis 127:388–393, 1973

205. Foz A, et al: *Mycobacterium chelonei* iatrogenic infections. J Clin Microbiol 7:319–321, 1978

206. France DR, Markham MP: Epidemiological aspects of *Proteus* infections with particular reference to phage typing. J Clin Pathol 21:97–102, 1968

207. Francis DP, et al: Nosocomial and maternally acquired *Herpesvirus hominis* infections. Am J Dis Child 129:889–893, 1975

208. Frank MJ, Schaffner W: Contaminated benzalkonium chloride. An unnecessary hospital infection hazard. JAMA 236:2418–2419, 1976

209. Freeman R, King B: Isolations of aerobic sporing bacilli from the tips of indwelling intravascular catheters. J Clin Pathol 28:146–148, 1975

210. Frommell GT, Bruhn FW, Schwartzman JD: Isolation of *Chlamydia trachomatis* from infant lung tissue. N Engl J Med 296:1150–1152, 1977

211. Fuchs PC: Indwelling intravenous polyethylene catheters: factors influencing the risk of microbial colonization and sepsis. JAMA 216:1447–1450, 1971

212. Fuchs PC: The replicator method for identification and biotyping of common bacterial isolates. Lab Med 6(No. 5):6–11, 1975

213. Gage AA, Dean DC, Schimert G, Minsley N: *Aspergillus* infection after cardiac surgery. Arch Surg 101:384–387, 1970

214. Gajdusek D, et al: Precautions in medical care of, and in handling materials from, patients with transmissible virus dementia (Creutzfeldt-Jakob disease). N Engl J Med 297:1253–1258, 1977

215. Gaman WJ, et al: Emergence of gentamicin and carbenicillin—resistant *Pseudomonas aeruginosa* in a hospital environment. Antimicrob Agents Chemother 9:474–480, 1976

216. Gangarosa EJ, Merson MH: Epidemiologic assessment of the relevance of the so-called enteropathogenic serogroups of *Escherichia coli* in diarrhea. N Engl J Med 296:1210–1213, 1977

217. Gantz NM, et al: Listerosis in immunosuppressed patients. A cluster of eight cases. Am J Med 58:637–643, 1975

218. Garb JL, Brown RB, Garb JR, Tuthill RW: Differences in etiology of pneumonias in nursing home and community patients. JAMA 240:2169–2172, 1978

219. Gardner P, Smith DH: Studies on the epidemiology of resistance (R) factors: I. Analysis of *Klebsiella* isolates in a general hospital, II. A prospective study of R factor transfer in the host. Ann Intern Med 71:1–9, 1969

220. Garfield MD, Ershler WB, Maki DG: Malaria transmission by platelet concentrate transfusion. JAMA 240:2285–2286, 1978

221. Garibaldi RA, et al: Hemodialysis—associated hepatitis. JAMA 225:384–389, 1973

222. Gartenberg G, Bottone EJ, Keusch GT, Weitzman I: Hospital-acquired mucormycosis (*Rhizopus rhizopodiformis*) of skin and subcutaneous tissue. N Engl J Med 299:1115–1118, 1978

223. Gelb AF, Seligman SJ: *Bacteroidaceae* bacteremia—effect of age and focus of infection upon clinical course. JAMA 212:1038–1041, 1970

224. George WL, et al: Aetiology of antimicrobial-agent-associated colitis. Lancet 1:802–803, 1978

225. Geraci JE, Forth RJ, Ellis FH: Postoperative prosthetic valve bacterial endocarditis due to *Corynebacterium xerosis*. Mayo Clin Proc 42:736–742, 1967

226. Gerner RE, Moore GE: BCG in cancer treatment. N Engl J Med 290:343, 1974

227. Ghamande AR, Landis FB, Snider GL: Bronchial geotrichosis with fungemia complicating bronchogenic carcinoma. Chest 59:98–101, 1971

228. Ghosal SP, et al: Noma neonatorum: its aetiopathogenesis. Lancet 2:289–291, 1978

229. Gifford RRM, Lambe DW, McElreath SD, Vogler WR: Septicemia due to *Aeromonas hydrophila* and *Mima polymorpha* in a patient with acute myelogenous leukemia. Am J Med Sci 263:157–161, 1972

230. Gilardi GL: *Pseudomonas maltophilia* infections in man. Am J Clin Pathol 51:58–61, 1969

231. Gilardi GL: Infrequently encountered *Pseudomonas* species causing infections in humans. Ann Intern Med 77:211–215, 1972

232. Gleason TH, Hamlin WB: Disseminated toxoplasmosis in the compromised host. A report of five cases. Arch Intern Med 134:1059–1062, 1974

233. Goffinet DR, Glatstein EJ, Merigan TC: Herpes zoster—varicella infections and lymphoma. Ann Intern Med 76:235-240, 1972

234. Glew RH, Buckley HR, Rosen HM, Moellering R Jr, Fischer JE: Serologic tests in the diagnosis of systemic candidiasis. Enhanced diagnostic accuracy with crossed immunoelectrophoresis. Am J Med 64:586-591, 1978

235. Goodman JS, Koenig MG: *Nocardia* infections in a general hospital. Ann NY Acad Sci 174:552-567, 1970

236. Gopal V, Bisno AL: Fulminant pneumococcal infections in "normal" asplenic hosts. Arch Intern Med 137:1526-1530, 1977

237. Gorbach SL, Thadepalli H: Isolation of *Clostridium* in human infections: evaluation of 114 cases. J Infect Dis 131(Supp):S81-S85, 1975

238. Govan JRW, Fyfe JAM: Mucoid *Pseudomonas aeruginosa* and cystic fibrosis: resistance of the mucoid form to carbenicillin, flucloxacillin, and tobramycin and the isolation of mucoid variants in vitro. J Antimicrob Chemother 4:233-240, 1978

239. Govan JRW, Gillies RR: Further studies in the pyocine typing of *Pseudomonas pyocyanea*. J Med Microbiol 2:17-25, 1969

240. Granoff DM, Nankervis A: Infectious arthritis in the neonate caused by *Haemophilus influenzae*. Am J Dis Child 129:730-733, 1975

241. Grant MD, Horowitz HI, Lorian V: Gangrenous ulcer and septicemia due to *Citrobacter*. N Engl J Med 280:1286-1287, 1969

242. Grant RM, et al: Results of administering BCG to patients with melanoma. Lancet 2:1096-1100, 1974

243. Gray RD, James SM: Occult diphtheria infection in a hospital for the mentally subnormal. Lancet 1:1105-1106, 1973

244. Grayston JT, Wang S: New knowledge of chlamydiae and the diseases they cause. J Infect Dis 132:87-105, 1975

245. Green GS, Johnson RH, Shively JA: Mimeae: opportunistic pathogens. JAMA 194:1065-1068, 1965

246. Green H, Macaulay MB: Hospital outbreak of *Listeria monocytogenes* septicemia: A problem of cross-infection? Lancet 2:1039-1040, 1978

247. Green SK, et al: Agricultural plants and soils as a reservoir for *Pseudomonas aeruginosa*. Appl Microbiol 28:987-991, 1974

248. Greene DC, Dodd MC: Recent developments in diarrhea of the newborn. NY State J Med 55:2764, 1955

249. Grieble HG, et al: Fine-particle humidifiers. Source of *Pseudomonas aeruginosa* infection in a respiratory-disease unit. N Engl J Med 282:531–535, 1970

250. Grist NR: Hepatitis in clinical laboratories. J Clin Pathol 31:415–417, 1978

251. Gross RJ, Rowe B, Easton JA: Neonatal meningitis caused by *Citrobacter koseri*. J Clin Pathol 26:138–139, 1973

252. Grossman J, Tompkins RL: Group B beta-hemolytic streptococcal meningitis in mother and infant. N Engl J Med 390:387–388, 1974

253. Gryska PF, O'Dea AE: Postoperative streptococcal wound infection. The anatomy of an epidemic. JAMA 213:1189–1191, 1970

254. Gullekson EH, Dumoff M: *Haemophilus parainfluenzae* meningitis in a newborn. JAMA 198:199, 1966

255. Gurwith MJ, Stinson EB, Remington JS: *Aspergillus* infection complicating cardiac transplantation. Arch Intern Med 128:541–545, 1971

256. Gwaltney JM, Moskalski PB, Hendley JO: Hand-to-hand transmission of rhinovirus colds. Ann Intern Med 88:463–467, 1978

257. Gwynn CM, George RH: Neonatal *Citrobacter* meningitis. Arch Dis Child 48:455–458, 1973

258. Hable KA, Horstmeier C, Wold AD, Washington JA II: Group A hemolytic streptococcemia. Bacteriologic and clinical study of 44 cases. Mayo Clin Proc 48:336–339, 1973

259. Hahn H, Condie F, Bulger RJ: Diagnosis of *Torulopsis glabrata* infection. Successful treatment of two cases. JAMA 203:835–837, 1968

260. Hall CB, Douglas G Jr, Geiman JM, Messner MK: Nosocomial respiratory syncytial virus infections. N Engl J Med 293:1343–1346, 1975

261. Hande KR, et al: Sepsis with a new species of *Corynebacterium*. Ann Intern Med 85:423–426, 1976

262. Handsfield HH, Hodson WA, Holmes KK: Neonatal gonococcal infection. I. Orogastric contamination with *Neisseria gonorrhoeae*. JAMA 225:697–701, 1973

263. Hanshaw JB: *Herpesvirus hominis* infections in the fetus and the newborn. Am J Dis Child 126:546–555, 1973

264. Hardy PC, Ederer GM, Matsen JM: Contamination of commercially packaged urinary catheter kits with the pseudomonad EO-1. N Engl J Med 282:33–35, 1970

265. Hare R, Thomas CGA: The transmission of *Staphylococcus aureus*. Br Med J 2:840–844, 1956

266. Harrison HR, English MG, Lee CK, Alexander ER: *C trachomatis* pneumonitis: comparison with matched infant controls and other pneumonitis. N Engl J Med 298:702–708, 1978

267. Hazuka BT, Dajani AS, Talbot K, Keen BH: Two outbreaks of *Flavobacterium meningosepticum* type E in a neonatal intensive care unit. J Clin Microbiol 6:450–455, 1977

268. Heathcote J, Cameron CH, Dane DS: Hepatitis-B antigen in saliva and semen. Lancet 1:71–73, 1974

269. Heckman MG, Babcock JB, Rose HD: Pyocine typing of *Pseudomonas aeruginosa*; clinical and epidemiologic aspects. Am J Clin Pathol 57:35–42, 1972

270. Hemming VG, McCloskey DW, Hill HR: Pneumonia in the neonate associated with group B streptococcal septicemia. Am J Dis Child 130:1231–1233, 1976

271. Henkel JS, Armstrong D, Blevins A, Moody MD: Group A β-hemolytic *Streptococcus* bacteremia in a cancer hospital. JAMA 211:983–986, 1970

272. Henle W, Henle GE, Horwitz CA: Epstein-Barr virus specific diagnostic tests in infectious mononucleosis. Hum Pathol 5:551–565, 1974

273. Henson D, et al: Cytomegalovirus infection during acute childhood leukemia. J Infect Dis 126:469–481, 1972

274. Herman LG, Himmelsbach CK: Detection and control of hospital sources of *Flavobacteria*. Hospitals 39:72–76, 1965

275. Hettiaratchy IGT, Cooke EM, Shooter RA: Colicine production as an epidemiological marker of *Escherichia coli*. J Med Microbiol 6:1–11, 1973

276. Hickman FW, Farmer JJ III: Differentiation of *Proteus mirabilis* by bacteriophage typing and the Dienes reaction. J Clin Microbiol 3:350–358, 1976

277. Hill J, Howell A, Blowers R: Effect of clothing on dispersal of *Staphylococcus aureus* by males and females. Lancet 2:1131–1133, 1974

278. Hill HR, et al: Epidemic of pharyngitis due to streptococci of Lancefield group G. Lancet 2:371–374, 1969

279. Hodges GR, Degener CE, Grindon AJ: Clinical significance of *Citrobacter* isolates. Am J Clin Pathol 70:37–40, 1978

280. Hoffmann PC, Dixon RE: Control of influenza in the hospital. Ann Intern Med 87:725–728, 1977

281. Holder IA, Kozinn PJ, Law EJ: Evaluation of *Candida* precipitin and agglutinin tests for the diagnosis of systemic candidiasis in burn patients. J Clin Microbiol 6:219-223, 1977

282. Hoofnagle JH, et al: Transmission of non-A, non-B hepatitis. Ann Intern Med 87:14-20, 1977

283. Howard FM, et al: Outbreak of necrotizing enterocolitis caused by *Clostridium butyricum*. Lancet 2:1099-1102, 1977

284. Hudson AW, McFarland C: Disseminated herpes simplex in a newborn: a consequence of infection in the mother. JAMA 208:859-861, 1969

285. Hughes RO: Hand, foot, and mouth disease associated with coxsackie A9 virus. Lancet 2:751-752, 1972

286. Hunt JS, et al: Granulomatous hepatitis: a complication of BCG immunotherapy. Lancet 2:820-821, 1973

287. Hurwich BJ: Monilial peritonitis. Arch Intern Med 117:405-408, 1966

288. Hyams PJ, et al: Staphylococcal bacteremia and hexachlorophene bathing. Epidemic in a newborn nursery. Am J Dis Child 129:595-599, 1975

289. Iannini PB, Claffey T, Quintiliani R: Bacteremic *Pseudomonas* pneumonia. JAMA 230:558-561, 1974

290. Iannini PB, Eickhoff TC, LaForce FM: Multidrug-resistant *Proteus rettgeri*: An emerging problem. Ann Intern Med 85:161-164, 1976

291. Ihde DC, Armstrong D: Clinical spectrum of infection due to *Bacillus* species. Am J Med 55:839-845, 1973

292. Isiadinso OA: *Listeria* sepsis and meningitis: a complication of renal transplantation. JAMA 234:842-843, 1975

293. Jackson GG, Muldoon RL: Viruses causing common respiratory infections in man. II. Enteroviruses and paramyxoviruses. J Infect Dis 128:387-469, 1973

294. Jackson GG, Muldoon RL: Viruses causing common respiratory infections in man. III. Respiratory syncytial viruses and coronaviruses. J Infect Dis 128:674-702, 1973

295. Jacobson RJ, et al: *Listeria* infections after splenectomy. N Engl J Med 287:721, 1972

296. Jahn CL, Cherry JD: Mild neonatal illness associated with heavy enterovirus infection. N Engl J Med 274:394-395, 1966

297. Janzen J, et al: Epidemiology of hepatitis B surface antigen (HB$_s$Ag) and antibody to HB$_s$Ag in hospital personnel. J Infect Dis 137:261-265, 1978

298. Jewett JF, Reid DE, Safon LE, Easterday CL: Childhood fever—a continuing entity. JAMA 206:344–350, 1968

299. Johanson WG, Pierce AM, Sanford JP: Changing pharyngeal flora of hospitalized patients. Emergence of gram-negative bacilli. N Engl J Med 281:1137–1140, 1969

300. Johanson WG Jr, Pierce AK, Sanford JP, Thomas GD: Nosocomial respiratory tract infections with gram-negative bacilli. The significance of colonization of the respiratory tract. Ann Intern Med 77:701–706, 1972

301. Johnson ML, Colley EW: *Listeria monocytogenes* encephalitis associated with corticosteroid therapy. J Clin Pathol 22:465–469, 1969

302. Johnson WD, Cobbs CG, Arditi LI, Kaye D: Diphtheroid endocarditis after insertion of a prosthetic heart valve. Report of two cases. JAMA 203:919–921, 1968

303. Jones RN, Slepack J: Fatal neonatal meningococcal meningitis. Association with maternal cervical-vaginal colonization. JAMA 236:2652–2653, 1976

304. Jones SR, Ragsdale AR, Kutscher E, Sanford JP: Clinical and bacteriological observations on a recently recognized species of Enterobacteriaceae, *Citrobacter diversus*. J Infect Dis 128:563–565, 1973

305. Jordan GW, Hadley WK: Human infection with *Edwardsiella tarda*. Ann Intern Med 70:283–288, 1969

306. Kagnoff MF, Armstrong D, Blevins A: *Bacteroides* bacteremia: experience in a hospital for neoplastic diseases. Cancer 29:245–251, 1972

307. Kaiser AB, et al: Antibiotic and antiseptic prophylaxis in vascular surgery. Ann Surg 188:283–289, 1978

308. Kammer RB, Utz JP: *Aspergillus* species endocarditis—the new face of a not so rare disease. Am J Med 56:506–521, 1974

309. Kane RC, et al: Cytomegalovirus infection in a volunteer blood donor population. Infect Immun 11:719–723, 1975

310. Kantor GL, Johnson BL Jr: Cytomegalovirus infection associated with cardiopulmonary bypass. Arch Intern Med 125:488–492, 1970

311. Kaplan MH, Armstrong D, Rosen P: Tuberculosis complicating neoplastic disease. Cancer 33:850–858, 1974

312. Kaplan K, Weinstein L: Diphtheroid infections of man. Ann Intern Med 70:919–929, 1969

313. Kaplan MH, Rosen PP, Armstrong D: Cryptococcosis in a cancer hospital. Clinical and pathological correlation in forty-six patients. Cancer 39:2265–2274, 1977

314. Karpas CM, Boman I: The significance of *Klebsiella* enteritis. Am J Clin Pathol 46:632–640, 1966

315. Kashbur IM, George RH, Ayliffe GAJ: Resistotyping of *Proteus mirabilis* and a comparison with other typing methods. J Clin Pathol 27:572–577, 1974

316. Kaslow RA, et al: Staphylococcal disease related to hospital nursery bathing practices—a nationwide epidemiologic investigation. Pediatrics 51:418–425, 1973

317. Kaslow RA, Mackel DC, Mallison GF: Nosocomial pseudobacteremia. Positive blood cultures due to contaminated benzalkonium antiseptic. JAMA 236:2407–2409, 1976

318. Kasper DL, et al: Isolation and identification of encapsulated strain of *Bacteroides fragilis*. J Infect Dis 136:75–81, 1977

319. Kass EH: Antimicrobial drug usage in general hospitals in Pennsylvania. Ann Intern Med 89:800–801, 1978

320. Kass EH, Schneiderman LJ: Entry of bacteria into the urinary tracts of patients with inlying catheters. N Engl J Med 256:556, 1957

321. Katzenstein A, Davis C, Braude A: Pulmonary changes in neonatal sepsis due to group B β-hemolytic *Streptococcus*: relation to hyaline membrane disease. J Infect Dis 133:430–435, 1976

322. Kauffman CA, Tan JS: *Torulopsis glabrata* renal infection. Am J Med 57:217–224, 1974

323. Kaufman SM: *Curvularia* endocarditis following cardiac surgery. Am J Clin Pathol 56:466–470, 1971

324. Kay JH, et al: Surgical treatment of *Candida* endocarditis. JAMA 203:621–626, 1968

325. Keane CT, English LF, Wise R: *Providencia stuartii* infections. Lancet 2:1045, 1975

326. Keene JK, et al: Disseminated varicella complicating ulcerative colitis. JAMA 239:45–46, 1978

327. Kennedy DH, et al: An outbreak of infantile gastroenteritis due to *E coli* 0142. J Clin Pathol 26:731–737, 1973

328. Khuri-Bulos N, McIntosh K: Neonatal *Haemophilis influenzae* infection. Am J Dis Child 129:57–62, 1975

329. Kilbourn JP: *Streptococcus pneumoniae* in chronic bronchitis. Lancet 1:1009, 1973

330. Kirby BD, Snyder KM, Meyer RD, Finegold SM: Legionnaires' disease: clinical features of 24 cases. Ann Intern Med 89:297-309, 1978

331. Kirmani N, et al: *Staphylococcus aureus* carriage rate of patients receiving long-term hemodialysis. Arch Intern Med 138:1657-1659, 1978

332. Klein JO, Buckland D, Finland M: Colonization of newborn infants by Mycoplasmas. N Engl J Med 280:1025-1030, 1969

333. Klimen JJ, et al: Clinical, epidemiologic and bacteriologic observations of an outbreak of methicillin-resistant *Staphylococcus aureus* at a large community hospital. Am J Med 61:341-345, 1976

334. Kominos SD, Copeland CE, Grosiak B: Mode of transmission of *Pseudomonas aeruginosa* in a burn unit and an intensive care unit in a general hospital. Appl Microbiol 23:309-312, 1972

335. Koopman JS, Campbell J: The role of cutaneous diphtheria infections in a diphtheria epidemic. J Infect Dis 131:239-244, 1975

336. Kraut MS, Attebery HR, Finegold SM, Sutter VL: Detection of *Haemophilus aphrophilus* in the human oral flora with a selective medium. J Infect Dis 126:189-192, 1972

337. Krick JA, Stinson EB, Remington JS: Nocardia infection in heart transplant patients. Ann Intern Med 82:18-26, 1975

338. Krogstad DJ, et al: Amebiosis: epidemiologic studies in the United States, 1971-1974. Ann Intern Med 88:89-97, 1978

339. Kulczyck LL, Murphy TM, Bellanti JA: *Pseudomonas* colonization in cystic fibrosis. A study of 160 patients. JAMA 240:30-34, 1978

340. Kurtz JB, Lee TW, Pickering D: Astrovirus associated gastroenteritis in a children's ward. J Clin Pathol 30:948-952, 1977

341. Kurup VP, Sheth NK: Immunotyping and pyocin typing of *Pseudomonas aeruginosa* from clinical specimens. Am J Clin Pathol 65:557-563, 1976

342. Kwon-Chung KJ, Young RC, Orlando M: Pulmonary mucormycosis caused by *Cunninghamella elegans* in a patient with chronic myelogenous leukemia. Am J Clin Pathol 64:544-548, 1975

343. Lacey RW: A critical appraisal of the importance of R-factors in the enterobacteriaceae *in vivo*. J Antimicrob Chemother 1:25-37, 1975

344. LaForce FM, Young LS, Bennett JV: Tetanus in the United States (1965-1966). Epidemiological and clinical factors. N Engl J Med 280:569-574, 1969

345. Langenhuysen MMAC, et al: Antibodies to Epstein-Barr virus, cytomegalovirus, and Australia antigens in Hodgkin's disease. Cancer 34:262–267, 1974

346. Larson HE, Price AB: Pseudomembranous colitis: presence of clostridial toxin. Lancet 2:1312–1314, 1977

347. Larson HE, Price RB, Honour P, Borriello SP: *Clostridium difficile* and the aetiology of pseudomembranous colitis. Lancet 1:1063–1066, 1978

348. Lautrop H: *Aeromonas hydrophila* isolated from human feces and its possible pathological significance. Acta Pathol Microbiol Scand 51 (suppl) 144:299–301, 1961

349. Lawrence T, Shockman AT, MacVaugh H: *Aspergillus* infection of prosthetic aortic valves. Chest 60:406–414, 1971

350. Ledger WJ: Hospital infections: gynecologic, obstetric, and perinatal infections. Ann Intern Med 89:774–776, 1978

351. Ledger WJ, Sweet RL, Headington JT: Prophylactic cephaloridine in the prevention of postoperative pelvic infections in premenopausal women undergoing vaginal hysterectomy. Am J Obstet Gynecol 115:766–774, 1973

352. Lee Y, et al: Wound infection with *Mycoplasma hominis*. JAMA 218:252–253, 1971

353. Leeber DA, Scher I: *Rhodotorula* fungemia presenting as "endotoxic" shock. Arch Intern Med 123:78–81, 1969

354. Leffert HL, Baptist JN, Gidez LI: Meningitis and bacteremia after ventriculoatrial shunt revision: isolation of a lecithinase-producing *Bacillus cereus*. J Infect Dis 122:547–552, 1970

355. Lehman TJA, Quinn JJ, Siegel SE, Ortega JA: *Clostridium septicum* infection in childhood leukemia. Report of a case and review of the literature. Cancer 40:950–953, 1972

356. Lerner PI, et al: Group B *Streptococcus* (*S agalactiae*) bacteremia in adults: analysis of 32 cases and review of the literature. Medicine 56:457–473, 1977

357. Levine MM, et al: *Escherichia coli* strains that cause diarrhea, but do not produce heat-labile or heat-stable enterotoxins and are non-invasive. Lancet 1:1119–1122, 1978

358. Levine MM, DuPont HL, Khodabandelou M, Hornick RB: Long-term shigella-carrier state. N Engl J Med 288:1169–1171, 1973

359. Levine PH, et al: Infectious mononucleosis prior to acute leukemia: A possible role for the Epstein-Barr virus. Cancer 30:875–880, 1972

360. Levy HL, O'Connor JF, Ingall D: Neonatal osteomyelitis due to *Proteus mirabilis*. JAMA 202:582–586, 1967

361. Lewis TL, et al: A comparison of the frequency of hepatitis-B antigen and antibody in hospital and non-hospital personnel. N Engl J Med 289:647–651, 1973

362. Light IJ, Sutherland JM, Cochran ML, Sutorius J: Ecologic relation between *Staphylococcus aureus* and *Pseudomonas* in a nursery population. N Engl J Med 278:1243–1247, 1968

363. Liljedahl SO, Malmborg AS, Nystrom B, Sjöberg L: Spread of *Pseudomonas aeruginosa* in a burn unit. J Med Microbiol 5:473–481, 1972

364. Linnemann CC Jr, Hegg ME, Ramundo N, Schiff GM: Screening hospital patients for hepatitis B surface antigen. Am J Clin Pathol 67:257–259, 1977

365. Lintz D, et al: Nosocomial *Salmonella* epidemic. Arch Intern Med 136:968–973, 1976

366. Liu PV: Changes in somatic antigens of *Pseudomonas aeruginosa* induced by bacteriophages. J Infect Dis 119:237–246, 1969

367. Lloyd-Still JD, Peter G, Lovejoy FH Jr: Infected "scalp-vein" needles. JAMA 213:1496–1497, 1970

368. Logan L: Atypical mycobacteria: Their clinical, laboratory and epidemiologic significance. Medicine 49:243–255, 1970

369. Lohr DC, Goeken JA, Doty DB, Donta ST: *Mycobacterium gordonae* infection of a prosthetic aortic valve. JAMA 239:1528–1530, 1978

370. London WT, et al: An epidemic of hepatitis in a chronic-hemodialysis unit. Australia antigen and differences in host response. N Engl J Med 281:571–578, 1969

371. Lopez JF, Quesada J, Saied A: Bacteremia and osteomyelitis due to *Aeromonas hydrophila*—a complication during the treatment of acute leukemia. Am J Clin Pathol 50:587–591, 1968

372. Louria DB, et al: Listerosis complicating malignant disease: a new association. Ann Intern Med 67:261–281, 1967

373. Lovrekovich L, Lovrekovich H, Jenkins DC: Use of ultraviolet light in the typing of *Pseudomonas aeruginosa* strains by pyocin production. J Clin Pathol 25:94–95, 1972

374. Lowbury EJL, Rabb JR, Roe E: Clearance from a hospital of gram-negative bacilli that transfer carbenicillin-resistance to *Pseudomonas aeruginosa*. Lancet 2:941–945, 1972

375. Lowbury EJL, et al: Sources of infection with *Pseudomonas aeruginosa* in patients with tracheostomy. J Med Microbiol 3:39–56, 1970

376. Lowenbraun S, et al: Infection from intravenous "scalp-vein" needles in a susceptible population. JAMA 212:451–453, 1970

377. Macasaet FF, Holley KE, Smith TF, Keys TF: Cytomegalovirus studies of autopsy tissue. II. Incidence of inclusion bodies and related pathologic data. Am J Clin Pathol 63:859–865, 1975

378. MacGregor RR, Reinhart J: Person-to-person spread of *Salmonella*: a problem in hospitals? Lancet 2:1001–1003, 1973

379. Madhavan T, Eisses J, Quinn EL: Infections due to *Trichosporon cutaneum*, an uncommon systemic pathogen. Henry Ford Hosp Med J 24:27–30, 1976

380. Madruga M, Zanon U, Pereira GMN, Galvao AC: Meningitis caused by *Flavobacterium meningosepticum*. The first epidemic outbreak of meningitis in the newborn in South America. J Infect Dis 121:328–330, 1970

381. Maki DG: Control of colonization and transmission of pathogenic bacteria in the hospital. Ann Intern Med 89:777–780, 1978

382. Maki DG, Goldmann DA, Rhame FS: Infection control in intravenous therapy. Ann Intern Med 79:867–887, 1973

383. Maki DG, et al: Nosocomial urinary tract infection with *Serratia marcescens*: An epidemiologic study. J Infect Dis 128:579–587, 1973

384. Marks MI, Langston C, Eickhoff TC: *Torulopsis glabrata*—an opportunistic pathogen in man. N Engl J Med 283:1131–1135, 1970

385. Martin WJ, Yu PKW, Washington JA II: Epidemiologic significance of *Klebsiella pneumoniae*—a 3-month study. Mayo Clin Proc 46:785–793, 1971

386. Masur H, Rosen PP, Armstrong D: Pulmonary disease caused by *Candida* species. Am J Med 63:914–925, 1977

387. Matsuda S, Tada K, Shirachi R, Ishida N: Australia antigen in amniotic fluid. Lancet 1:1117, 1972

388. Mazur MH, Dolin R: Herpes zoster at the NIH: A 20 year experience. Am J Med 65:738–744, 1978

389. McCormack WM, et al: Vaginal colonization with *Corynebacterium vaginale* (*Haemophilus vaginalis*). J Infect Dis 136:740–745, 1977

390. McCormack WM, et al: Isolation of genital Mycoplasmas from blood obtained shortly after vaginal delivery. Lancet 1:596–599, 1975

391. McCracken GH Jr, et al: Relation between *Escherichia coli* KI capsular polysaccharide antigen and clinical outcome in neonatal meningitis. Lancet 2:246–250, 1974

392. McGowan JE Jr, Finland M: Usage of antibiotics in a general hospital: effect of requiring justification. J Infect Dis 130:165–168, 1974

393. McKee WM, DiCaprio JM, Roberts CE Jr, Sherris JC: Anal carriage as a probable source of streptococcal epidemic. Lancet 2:1007–1009, 1966

394. McLeish WA, Elder RH, Westwood JCN: Contaminated vacuum tubes. (Letter) Can Med Assoc J 112:682, 1975

395. McRae AT, Pate JW, Richardson RL: Aortic valve replacement for *Candida* endocarditis. Chest 62:757–758, 1972

396. Meadow SR, Weller RO, Archibald RWR: Fatal systemic measles in a child receiving cyclophosphamide for nephrotic syndrome. Lancet 2:876–878, 1969

397. Meltz DJ, Grieco MH: Characteristics of *Serratia marcescens* pneumonia. Arch Intern Med 132:359–364, 1973

398. Meyer RD, Rosen P, Armstrong D: Phycomycosis complicating leukemia and lymphoma. Ann Intern Med 77:871–879, 1972

399. Meyer RD, Young LS, Armstrong D, Yu B: Aspergillosis complicating neoplastic disease. Am J Med 54:6–15, 1973

400. Meyers BR, Bottone E, Hirschman SZ, Schneierson SS: Infections caused by microorganisms of the genus *Erwinia*. Ann Intern Med 76:9–14, 1972

401. Meyers JD, et al: Parenterally transmitted non-A, non-B hepatitis: an epidemic reassessed. Ann Intern Med 87:57–59, 1977

402 Meyers JD, et al: Parenterally transmitted hepatitis A associated with platelet transfusions. Epidemiologic study of an outbreak in a marrow transplantation center. Ann Intern Med 81:145–151, 1974

403. Meyers JD, Romm FJ, Tihen WS, Bryan JA: Foodborne hepatitis A in a general hospital. Epidemiologic study of an outbreak attributed to sandwiches. JAMA 231:1049–1053, 1975

404. Meyers JD, et al: Cytomegalovirus pneumonia after human bone marrow transplantation. Ann Intern Med 82:181–188, 1975

405. Meyers JD, Stamm WE, Kerr MM, Counts GW: Lack of transmission of hepatitis B after surgical exposure. JAMA 240:1725–1727, 1978

406. Miller G: The oncogenicity of Epstein-Barr virus. J Infect Dis 130:187–205, 1974

407. Miller JK, Hedberg M: Effects of cortisone on susceptibility of mice to *Listeria monocytogenes*. Am J Clin Pathol 43:248–250, 1965

408. Millian SJ, Baldwin JN, Rheins MS, Weiser HH: Studies on the incidence of coagulase-positive staphylococci in a normal unconfined population. Am J Public Health 50:791–798, 1960

409. Mills CC: Occurrence of *Mycobacterium* other than *Mycobacterium tuberculosis* in the oral cavity and in sputum. Appl Microbiol 24:307–310, 1972

410. Mirkovic R, Werch J, South MA, Benyesh-Melnick M: Incidence of cytomegaloviremia in blood-bank donors and in infants with congenital cytomegalic inclusion disease. Infect Immun 3:45–50, 1971

411. Mitchell RG, Guillebaud J, Day DG: Group B streptococci in women fitted with intrauterine devices. J Clin Pathol 30:1021–1024, 1977

412. Montgomerie JZ, et al: Herpes-simplex virus infection after renal transplantation. Lancet 2:867–871, 1969

413. Montgomerie JZ, et al: *Klebsiella* in fecal flora of renal transplant patients. Lancet 2:787–791, 1970

414. Moody MR, Young VM, Kenton DM, Vermeulen GD: *Pseudomonas aeruginosa* in a center for cancer research. I. Distribution of intraspecies types from human and environmental sources. J Infect Dis 125:95–101, 1972

415. Moore B, Forman A: An outbreak of urinary *Pseudomonas aeruginosa* infection acquired during urological operations. Lancet 2:929–931, 1966

416. Morehead CD, Houck PW: Epidemiology of *Pseudomonas* infection in a pediatric intensive care unit. Am J Dis Child 124:564–570, 1972

417. Morse LJ, et al: Septicemia due to *Klebsiella pneumoniae* from a hand-cream dispenser. N Engl J Med 277:472–473, 1967

418. Muller SA, Herrmann EC Jr, Winkelmann RK: Herpes simplex infections in hematologic malignancies. Am J Med 52:102–114, 1972

419. Mummery RV, Rowe B, Gross RJ: Urinary tract infections due to atypical *Enterobacter cloacae*. Lancet 2:1333, 1974

420. Musher DM, McKenzie SO: Infections due to *Staphylococcus aureus*. Medicine 56:383–409, 1977

421. Myerowitz RL, Pazin GJ, Allen CM: Disseminated candidiasis: changes in incidence, underlying diseases and pathology. Am J Clin Pathol 68:29–38, 1977

422. Myers MG, McMahon BJ, Koontz FP: Neonatal calcaneous osteomyelitis related to contaminated mineral oil. J Clin Microbiol 6:543–544, 1977

423. Nagington J, et al: Fatal echovirus 11 infection in outbreak in special-care baby unit. Lancet 2:725–728, 1978

424. Nahmias AJ, Godwin JT, Updyke EL, Hopkins WA: Post-surgical staphylococcal infections. Outbreak traced to an individual carrying phage strain 80/81 and 80/81/52/52A. JAMA 174:1269–1275, 1960

425. Nahmias AJ, Josey WE, Naib ZM: Neonatal herpes simplex infection. Role of genital infection in mother as source of virus in the newborn. JAMA 199:164–168, 1967

426. Najem GR, Riley HD, Ordway NK, Yoshioka H: Clinical and microbiological surveillance of neonatal staphylococcal disease. Relationship to hexachlorophene whole-body bathing. Am J Dis Child 129:297–302, 1975

427. Naraqi S, Jackson GG, Jonasson OM: Viremia with herpes simplex type I in adults: four nonfatal cases, one with features of chicken pox. Ann Intern Med 85:165–169, 1976

428. Naraqi S, Jackson GG, Jonasson O, Yamashiroya HM: Prospective study of prevalence, incidence and source of herpesvirus infections in patients with renal allografts. J Infect Dis 136:531–540, 1977

429. Nash G, et al: Fungal burn wound infection. JAMA 215:1664–1666, 1971

430. Nathan P, Holder IA, MacMillan BG: Burn wounds: microbiology, local host defenses, and current therapy. Crit Rev Clin Lab Sci 4:61–100, 1973

431. Neary MP, Allen J, Okubadejo OA, Payne DJH: Preoperative vaginal bacteria and postoperative infections in gynecological patients. Lancet 2:1291–1294, 1973

432. Neefe LI, Pinilla O, Garagusi VF, Bauer H: Disseminated strongyloidiasis with cerebral involvement. A complication of corticosteroid therapy. Am J Med 55:832–838, 1973

433. Neff JM, Lane JM: Vaccinia necrosum following smallpox vaccination for chronic herpetic ulcers. JAMA 213:123–125, 1970

434. Nelson DL, Hable KL, Matsen JM: *Proteus mirabilis* osteomyelitis in two neonates following needle puncture. Successful treatment with ampicillin. Am J Dis Child 125:109–110, 1973

435. Newsom SWB: Hospital infection from contaminated ice. Lancet 2:620–622, 1968

436. Niederman JC, et al: Infectious mononucleosis. Epstein-Barr-virus shedding in saliva and the oropharynx. N Engl J Med 294:1355–1359, 1976

437. Nieman PE, et al: A prospective analysis of interstitial pneumonia and opportunistic viral infection among recipients of allogenic bone marrow grafts. J Infect Dis 136:754–767, 1977

438. Nolan CM, Beaty HN: *Staphylococcus aureus* bacteremia. Current clinical patterns. Am J Med 60:495–500, 1976

439. Noone P, Griffiths RJ, Taylor CED: Hexachlorophene for treating carriers of *Staphylococcus aureus*. Lancet 1:1202–1203, 1970

440. Noone P, Rogers BT: Pneumonia caused by coliforms and *Pseudomonas aeruginosa*. J Clin Pathol 29:652–656, 1976

441. Oblack D, Schwartz J, Holder IA: Comparative evaluation of the *Candida* agglutinin test, precipitin test and germ tube dispersion test in the diagnosis of candidiasis. J Clin Microbiol 3:175–179, 1976

442. Odds FC, Evans EGV, Taylor HAR, Wales JK: Prevalence of pathogenic yeasts and humoral antibodies to *Candida* in diabetic patients. J Clin Pathol 31:840–844, 1978

443. Okada DM, Chow AW: Neonatal scalp abscess following intrapartum fetal monitoring: a prospective comparison of two spiral electrodes. Am J Obstet Gynecol 127:875–878, 1977

444. Olds JW, Kisch AL, Eberle BJ, Wilson JN: *Pseudomonas aeruginosa* respiratory tract infection acquired from a contaminated anesthesia machine. Am Rev Respir Dis 105:628–632, 1972

445. Olsen H: An epidemiological study of hospital infection with *Flavobacterium meningosepticum*. Dan Med Bull 14:6–9, 1967

446. Olsen H, Frederiksen WC, Siboni KE: *Flavobacterium meningosepticum* in 8 non-fatal cases of postoperative bacteremia. Lancet 1:1294–1296, 1965

447. Olsen H, Ravn T: *Flavobacterium meningosepticum* isolated from the genitals. Acta Pathol Microbiol Scand B 79:102–106, 1971

448. Onderdonk AB, Kasper DL, Cisneros RL, Bartlett JG: The capsular polysaccharide of *Bacteroides fragilis* as a virulence factor: comparison of the pathogenic potential of encapsulated and unencapsulated strains. J Infect Dis 136:82–89, 1977

449. Ortel S: Intrauterine listerosis infection, in Thalhammer O (ed): Prenatal Infections. New York: Grune & Stratton, Inc., pp. 1–8, 1971

450. O'Toole RD, Drew WL, Dahlgren BS, Beaty HN: An outbreak of methicillin-resistant *Staphylococcus aureus* infections. Observations in hospital and nursing home. JAMA 213:257–263, 1970

451. Overturf GD, Wilkins J, Ressler R: Emergence of resistance of *Providencia stuartii* to multiple antibiotics: speciation and biochemical characterization of *Providencia*. J Infect Dis 129:353–357, 1974

452. Page MI, King EO: Infection due to *Actinobacillus actinomycetemcommitans* and *Haemophilus aphrophilus*. N Engl J Med 275:181–188, 1966

453. Painter BG, Isenberg HD: Isolation of *Candida parapsilosis*: report of two cases. Am J Clin Pathol 59:62–65, 1973

454. Pankey GA, Daloviso JR: Fungemia caused by *Torulopsis glabrata*. Medicine 52:395–403, 1973

455. Paradinas FJ, Wiltshaw E: Necropsy findings in a case of progressive vaccinia. J Clin Pathol 25:233–239, 1972

456. Parker JC, McCloskey JJ, Knauer KA: Pathobiologic features of human candidiasis—a common deep mycosis of the brain, heart and kidney in the altered host. Am J Clin Pathol 65:991–1000, 1976

457. Parker MT, Ball LC: Streptococci and aerococci associated with systemic infections in man. J Med Microbiol 9:275–302, 1976

458. Parkhurst GF, Vlahides GD: Fatal opportunistic fungus disease. JAMA 202:279–281, 1967

459. Passwell J, et al: Fatal disseminated BCG infections. Am J Dis Child 130:433–436, 1976

460. Patterson MJ, Hafeel AEB: Group B streptococci in human disease. Bacteriol Rev 40:774–792, 1976

461. Pazin GJ, Ho M, Jannetta PJ: Reactivation of herpes simplex virus after decompression of the trigeminal nerve root. J Infect Dis 138:405–409, 1978

462. Pead L, Crump J, Maskell R: Staphylococci as urinary pathogens. J Clin Pathol 30:427–431, 1977

463. Pearson HE: Human infections caused by organisms of the *Bacillus* species. Am J Clin Pathol 53:506–515, 1970

464. Pearson TA, Braine HG, Rathbun HK: *Corynebacterium* sepsis in oncology patients: Predisposing factors, diagnosis and treatment. JAMA 238:1737–1740, 1977

465. Pearson TA, Mitchell CA, Hughes WT: *Aeromonas hydrophila* septicemia. Am J Dis Child 123:579–582, 1972

466. Pedersen MM, Marso E, Pickett MJ: Nonfermentative bacilli associated with man: III. Pathogenicity and antibiotic susceptibility. Am J Clin Pathol 54:178–192, 1970

467. Penner JL, Hinton NA, Hennessy J: Biotypes of *Proteus rettgeri*. J Clin Microbiol 1:136–142, 1975

468. Penner JL, Hinton NA, Hennessy JN: Evaluation of a *Proteus rettgeri* O-serotyping system for epidemiological investigation. J Clin Microbiol 3:385–389, 1976

469. Penner JL, Hinton NA, Whiteley GR, Hennessy JN: Variation in urease activity of endemic hospital strains of *Proteus rettgeri* and *Providencia stuartii*. J Infect Dis 134:370–376, 1976

470. Pennington JE, et al: *Bacillus* species infection in patients with hematologic neoplasia. JAMA 235:1473–1474, 1976

471. Pennington JE, Reynolds HY, Carbone PP: *Pseudomonas* pneumonia. A retrospective study of 36 cases. Am J Med 55:155–160, 1973

472. Perera DR, et al: *Pneumocystis carinii* pneumonia in a hospital for children: Epidemiologic aspects. JAMA 214:1074–1078, 1970

473. Peter G, Lloyd-Still JD, Lovejoy FH: Local infection and bacteremia from scalp vein needles and polyethylene catheters in children. J Pediatr 80:78–83, 1972

474. Petersen DL, Hudson LD, Sullivan K: Disseminated *Nocardia caviae* with positive blood cultures. Arch Intern Med 138:1164–1165, 1978

475. Phillips I, Eykyn S, Curtis MA, Snell JJS: *Pseudomonas cepacia* (multivorans) septicemia in an intensive-care unit. Lancet 1:375–377, 1971

476. Pien FD, Martin WJ, Hermans PE, Washington JA II: Clinical and bacteriologic observations on the proposed species. *Enterobacter agglomerans* (the *Herbricola lathyri* bacteria). Mayo Clin Proc 47:739–745, 1972

477. Pien FD, Thompson RL, Martin WJ: Clinical and bacteriological studies of anaerobic gram-positive cocci. Mayo Clin Proc 47:251–257, 1972

478. Plaut ME, et al: Staphylococcal bacteremia in a "germ-free" unit. Arch Intern Med 136:1238–1240, 1976

479. Plotkin SA, McKitrick JC: Nosocomial meningitis of the newborn caused by a *Flavobacterium*. JAMA 198:662–664, 1966

480. Plouffe JF, et al: Nosocomial outbreak of *Candida parapsilosis* fungemia related to intravenous infusions. Arch Intern Med 137:1686–1689, 1977

481. Polk HC: Prevention of surgical wound infections. Ann Intern Med 89:770–773, 1978

482. Pollack AA, Holzman RS: *Neisseria catarrhalis* endocarditis. Ann Intern Med 85:206–207, 1976

483. Pollack HM, Dahlgren BJ: Distribution of streptococcal groups in clinical specimens with evaluation of bacitracin screening. Appl Microbiol 27:141–143, 1974

484. Porschen RK, Chan P: Anaerobic vibrio-like organisms cultured from blood: *Desulfovibrio desulfuricans* and *Succinivibrio* species. J Clin Microbiol 5:444–447, 1977

485. Porschen RK, Goodman Z, Rafai B: Isolation of *Corynebacterium xerosis* from clinical specimens: Infection and colonization. Am J Clin Pathol 68:290–293, 1977

486. Price DJE, Sleigh JD: Control of infections due to *Klebsiella aerogenes* in a neurosurgical unit by withdrawal of all antibiotics. Lancet 2:1213–1215, 1970

487. Prince AM, et al: Long-incubation post-transfusion hepatitis without serological evidence of exposure to hepatitis-B virus. Lancet 2:241–246, 1974

488. Prince AM, Szmuness W, Millian SJ, David DS: A serologic study of cytomegalovirus infections associated with blood transfusions. N Engl J Med 284:1125–1131, 1971

489. Qadri SMH, Wende GRD, Williams RP: Meningitis due to *Aeromonas hydrophila*. J Clin Microbiol 3:102–104, 1976

490. Quintiliani R, Gifford RH: Endocarditis from *Serratia marcescens*. JAMA 208:2055–2059, 1969

491. Quirante J, Ceballos R, Cassady G: Group B β-hemolytic streptococcal infection in the newborn. Am J Dis Child 128:659–665, 1974

492. Rado JP, et al: Herpes zoster house epidemics in steroid-treated patients. Arch Intern Med 116:329–335, 1965

493. Rahal JJ Jr, Meade RH III, Bump CM, Reinauer AJ: Upper respiratory tract carriage of gram-negative enteric bacilli by hospital personnel. JAMA 214:754–756, 1970

494. Rakela J, Mosley JW: Fecal excretion of hepatitis A virus in humans. J Infect Dis 135:933–938, 1977

495. Rames L, Wise B, Goodman JR, Piel CF: Renal disease with *Staphylococcus albus* bacteremia. A complication in ventriculoatrial shunts. JAMA 212:1671–1677, 1970

496. Rand KH, Pollard RB, Merigan TC: Increased pulmonary superinfections in cardiac-transplant patients undergoing primary cytomegalovirus infection. N Engl J Med 298:951–953, 1978

497. Rand KH, et al: Cellular immunity and herpesvirus infections in cardiac-transplant patients. N Engl J Med 296:1372–1377, 1976

498. Rathbun HK: Clostridial bacteremia without hemolysis. Arch Intern Med 122:496–501, 1968

499. Reboul F, Donaldson SS, Kaplan HS: Herpes zoster and varicella infections in children with Hodgkin's disease. An analysis of contributing factors. Cancer 41:95–99, 1978

500. Regamey C, Schoenknecht FD: Puerperal fever with *Haemophilus vaginalis* sepsis. JAMA 225:1621–1623, 1973

501. Rennie RP, Duncan IBR: Combined biochemical and serological typing of clinical isolates of *Klebsiella*. Appl Microbiol 28:534–539, 1974

502. Reynolds ES, Walls KW, Pfeiffer RI: Generalized toxoplasmosis following renal transplantation. Report of a case. Arch Intern Med 118:401–405, 1966

503. Rhames FS, et al: *Salmonella* septicemia from platelet transfusions. Study of an outbreak traced to a hematogenous carrier of *Salmonella choleraesuis*. Ann Intern Med 78:633–641, 1973

504. Ribeiro CD, Davis P, Jones DM: *Citrobacter koseri* meningitis in a special care baby unit. J Clin Pathol 29:1094–1096, 1976

505. Richman LS, Short WF, Cooper WM: Barium enema septicemia: occurrence in a patient with leukemia. JAMA 226:62–63, 1973

506. Rifkind D, Faris TD, Hill RB Jr: *Pneumocystis carinii* pneumonia. Studies on the diagnosis and treatment. Ann Intern Med 65:943–956, 1966

507. Rifkin GD, Fekety FR, Silva J Jr, Sack RB: Antibiotic-induced colitis implication of a toxin neutralized by *Clostridium sordellii* antitoxin. Lancet 2:1103–1106, 1977

508. Ritch PS, McCredie KP, Gutterman JU, Hersh EM: Disseminated BCG disease associated with immunotherapy by scarification in acute leukemia. Cancer 42:167–170, 1978

509. Rivera E, et al: Hyperinfection syndrome with *Strongyloides stercoralis*. Ann Intern Med 72:199–204, 1970

510. Ringrose RE, et al: A hospital outbreak of *Serratia marcescens* associated with ultrasonic nebulizers. Ann Intern Med 69:719–729, 1968

511. Robbins JB, et al: *Escherichia coli* K1 capsular polysaccharide associated with neonatal meningitis. N Engl J Med 290:1216–1220, 1974

512. Robinson MG, Halpern C: Infections, *Escherichia coli*, and sickle cell anemia. JAMA 230:1145–1148, 1974

513. Roessmann U, Friede RL: Candidal infection of the brain. Arch Pathol 84:495–498, 1967

514. Rogers WA Jr, Nelson B: Strongyloidiasis and malignant lymphoma. "Opportunistic infection" by a nematode. JAMA 195:685–687, 1966

515. Roques D: Melioidose post-operatoire et localisation chirurgicale de la melioidose. Rev Med Franc d'Extreme-Orient 21:267–275, 1943

516. Rose HD, Koch ML: Hospital-acquired *Aerobacter cloacae* infections. Results of two concomitant studies. Arch Intern Med 117:92–98, 1966

517. Rose HD, Sheth NK: Pulmonary candidiasis. A clinical and pathological correlation. Arch Intern Med 138:964–965, 1978

518. Rosen P, Hajdu S: Cytomegalovirus inclusion disease at autopsy of patients with cancer. Am J Clin Pathol 55:749–756, 1971

519. Rosen P, Hajdu SI: Visceral herpesvirus infections in patients with cancer. Am J Clin Pathol 56:459–465, 1971

520. Rosenbaum EH, Cohen RA, Glatstein HR: Vaccination of a patient receiving immunosuppressive therapy for lymphosarcoma. JAMA 198:737–740, 1966

521. Rosenberg EB, Kanne SR, Schwartzman RJ, Colsky J: Systemic infection following BCG therapy. Arch Intern Med 134:769–770, 1974

522. Rosenberg JL, Jones DP, Lipitz LR, Kirsner JB: Viral hepatitis: an occupational hazard to surgeons. JAMA 223:395–400, 1973

523. Rosenberg SA, Seipp C, Sears HF: Clinical and immunological studies of disseminated BCG infection. Cancer 41:1771–1780, 1978

524. Roth JA, Siegel SE, Levine AS, Berard CW: Fatal recurrent toxoplasmosis in a patient initially infected via a leukocyte transfusion. Am J Clin Pathol 56:601–605, 1971

525. Rubin SJ, Brock S, Chamberland M, Lyons RW: Combined serotyping and biotyping of *Serratia marcescens*. J Clin Microbiol 3:582–585, 1976

526. Rubin SJ, Lyons RW, Murcia AJ: Endocarditis associated with cardiac catheterization due to a gram-positive coccus designated *Micrococcus muciloginosus incertae sedis*. J Clin Microbiol 7:546–549, 1978

527. Ruskin J, Remington JS: Toxoplasmosis in the compromised host. Ann Intern Med 84:193–199, 1976

528. Ryder RW, et al: Infantile diarrhea produced by heat-stable enterotoxigenic *Escherichia coli*. N Engl J Med 295:849–853, 1976

529. St Geme JW Jr, et al: Neonatal risk following late gestational genital *Herpesvirus hominis* infection. Am J Dis Child 129:342–343, 1975

530. Sande MA, Levinson ME, Lukas DS, Kaye D: Bacteremia associated with cardiac catheterization. N Engl J Med 281:1104–1106, 1969

531. Sanders CV, et al: *Serratia marcescens* infections from inhalation therapy medication: Nosocomial outbreak. Ann Intern Med 73:15–21, 1970

532. Sarff LD, et al: Epidemiology of *Escherichia coli* K1 in healthy and diseased newborns. Lancet 1:1099–1104, 1975

533. Saunders AM, Bieber C: Pathologic findings in a case of cardiac transplantation. JAMA 206:815–820, 1968

534. Schaberg DR, et al: An outbreak of nosocomial infection due to multiply resistant *Serratia marcescens*: Evidence of inter-hospital spread. J Infect Dis 134:181–188, 1976

535. Schaffner W, Lefkowitz LB Jr, Goodman JS, Koenig MG: Hospital outbreak of infections with group A streptococci traced to an asymptomatic anal carrier. N Engl J Med 280:1224–1225, 1969

536. Schaffner W, Reisig G, Verrall RA: Outbreak of *Pseudomonas cepacia* infection due to contaminated anesthetics. Lancet 1:1050–1051, 1973

537. Scheckler WE: Septicemia and nosocomial infections in a community hospital. Ann Intern Med 89:754–756, 1978

538. Schimpff S, et al: Varicella-zoster infections in patients with cancer. Ann Intern Med 76:241–254, 1972

539. Schimpff SC, et al: Origin of infection in acute nonlymphocytic leukemia. Significance of hospital acquisition of potential pathogens. Ann Intern Med 77:707–714, 1972

540. Schmidt WC, Jeffries CD: Bacteriophage typing of *Proteus mirabilis*, *Proteus vulgaris*, and *Proteus morgani*. Appl Microbiol 27:47–53, 1974

541. Schroeder SA, Aserkoff B, Brachman PS: Epidemic salmonellosis in hospitals and institutions—a five year review. N Engl J Med 279:674–678, 1968

542. Schwarzmann SW, et al: Bacterial pneumonia during the Hong Kong influenza epidemic of 1968-1969. Arch Intern Med 127:1037–1041, 1971

543. Scott JM, Henderson A: Acute villous inflammation in the placenta following intrauterine transfusion. J Clin Pathol 25:872–875, 1972

544. Scowden EB, Schaffner W, Stone WJ: Overwhelming strongyloidiasis. Medicine 57:527–544, 1978

545. Scully RE, Galdabini JJ, McNeely BU (eds): Case records of the Massachusetts General Hospital. N Engl J Med 293:443–448, 1975

546. Seeler RA, Metzger W, Mufson MA: *Diplococcus pneumoniae* infections in children with sickle cell anemia. Am J Dis Child 123:8–10, 1972

547. Seeler RA, Miller RA, Lin C, Lin S: Transfusion-induced malaria. *Plasmodium vivax* in a 5-month old child. Am J Dis Child 125:132-133, 1973

548. Selden R, et al: Nosocomial *Klebsiella* infections: Intestinal colonization as a reservoir. Ann Intern Med 74:657-664, 1971

549. Semel JD, et al: *Pseudomonas maltophilia* pseudosepticemia. Am J Med 64:403-406, 1978

550. Senior BW: Typing of *Proteus* species by proticine production and sensitivity. J Med Microbiol 10:7-17, 1977

551. Sexton DJ, et al: Amebiasis in a mental institution: serologic and epidemiologic studies. Am J Epidemiol 100:414-423, 1974

552. Sharpe ME, Hill LR, Lapage SP: Pathogenic lactobacilli. J Med Microbiol 6:281-286, 1973

553. Sherman JD, Ingall D, Wiener J, Pryles CV: *Alcaligenes faecalis* infection in the newborn. Am J Dis Child 100:212-216, 1960

554. Shikata T, et al: Hepatitis B e antigen and infectivity of hepatitis B virus. J Infect Dis 136:571-576, 1977

555. Shirachi R, et al: Hepatitis "C" antigen in non-A, non-B post-transfusion hepatitis. Lancet 2:853-856, 1978

556. Shooter RA, et al: Food and medicaments as possible sources of hospital strains of *Pseudomonas aeruginosa*. Lancet 1:1227-1229, 1969

557. Shooter RA, Cooke EM, Rousseau SA, Breaden AL: Animal sources of common serotypes of *Escherichia coli* in the food of hospital patients. Possible significance in urinary tract infections. Lancet 2:226-228, 1970

558. Shooter RA, et al: Isolation of *Escherichia coli*, *Pseudomonas aeruginosa* and *Klebsiella* from food in hospitals, canteens, and schools. Lancet 2:390-392, 1971

559. Shooter RA, Stoodley BJ, Gordon B: Control of an outbreak of sepsis due to *Staphylococcus aureus* phage-type 52/52A/80/81, in nurses. Lancet 1:293-295, 1968

560. Shooter RA, et al: Faecal carriage of *Pseudomonas aeruginosa* in hospital patients. Possible spread from patient to patient. Lancet 2:1331-1334, 1966

561. Shortland-Webb WR: *Proteus* and coliform meningoencephalitis in neonates. J Clin Pathol 21:422-431, 1968

562. Simberkoff MS, Toharsky B: Mycoplasmemia in adult male patients. JAMA 236:2522-2524, 1976

Hospital–Associated Infections

563. Simon G, von Graevenitz A: Intestinal and water-borne infections due to *Aeromonas hydrophila*. Public Health Lab 27:159–162, 1969

564. Simpson MB Jr, Merz WG, Kurlinski JP, Solomon MH: Opportunistic mycotic osteomyelitis: Bone infections due to *Aspergillus* and *Candida* species. Medicine 56:475–482, 1977

565. Singer C, Armstrong D, Rosen PP, Schottenfeld D: *Pneumocystis carinii* pneumonia: A cluster of eleven cases. Ann Intern Med 82:772–777, 1975

566. Sinkovics JG, Smith JP: Septicemia and *Bacteroides* in patients with malignant disease. Cancer 25:663–671, 1970

567. Skirrow MB: The Dienes (mutual inhibition) test in the investigation of *Proteus* infections. J Med Microbiol 2:471–477, 1969

568. Smit P, et al: Protective efficacy of pneumococcal polysaccharide vaccines. JAMA 238:2613–2616, 1977

569. Smith JA, O'Connor JJ, Willis AT: Nasal carriage of *Staphylococcus aureus* in diabetes mellitus. Lancet 2:776–777, 1966

570. Smith JB, et al: Multicystic cerebral degeneration in neonatal herpes-simplex virus encephalitis. Am J Dis Child 131:568–572, 1977

571. Smith PW, Massanari RM: Room humidifiers as the source of *Acinetobacter* infections. JAMA 237:795–797, 1977

572. Smith RF, Blasi D, Dayton SL: Isolation and characterization of corynebacteria from burned children. Appl Microbiol 26:554–559, 1973

573. Smith RF, Dayton SL, Chipps DD: Autograft rejection in acutely burned patients: Relation to colonization by *Streptococcus agalactiae*. Appl Microbiol 25:493–495, 1973

574. Snydman DR, Bryan JA, Dixon RE: Prevention of nosocomial viral hepatitis, type B (hepatitis B). Ann Intern Med 83:838–845, 1975

575. Solberg CO, Matsen JM: Infections with *Providencia* bacilli. A clinical and bacteriologic study. Am J Med 50:241–246, 1971

576. Spector D: Hepatitis B miniepidemic in a peritoneal dialysis unit. Arch Intern Med 137:1030–1031, 1977

577. Speers R Jr, et al: Contamination of nurses' uniforms with *Staphylococcus aureus*. Lancet 2:233–235, 1969

578. Speller DCE, Mitchell RG: Coagulase-negative staphylococci causing endocarditis after cardiac surgery. J Clin Pathol 26:517–527, 1973

579. Speller DCE, et al: Epidemic infection by a gentamicin-resistant *Staphylococcus aureus* in three hospitals. Lancet 1:464–466, 1976

580. Spencer AG, et al: *Escherichia coli* serotypes in urinary-tract infections in a medical ward. Lancet 2:839–842, 1968

581. Spengler RF, Greenbough WB: Hospital costs and mortality attributed to nosocomial bacteremias. JAMA 240:2455–2458, 1978

582. Stamm WE: Infection related to medical devices. Ann Intern Med 89:764–769, 1978

583. Stamm WE, Colella JJ, Anderson RL, Dixon RE: Indwelling arterial catheters as a source of nosocomial bacteremia. An outbreak caused by *Flavobacterium* species. N Engl J Med 292:1099–1102, 1975

584. Stamm WE, Feeley JC, Facklam RR: Wound infections due to group A *Streptococcus* traced to a vaginal carrier. J Infect Dis 138:287–292, 1978

585. Stanton RE, Lindesmith GG, Meyer BW: *Escherichia coli* endocarditis after repair of ventricular septal defect. N Engl J Med 279:737–742, 1968

586. Steere AC, et al: Person-to-person spread of *Salmonella typhimurium* after a hospital common-source outbreak. Lancet 1:319–322, 1975

587. Steere AC, et al: *Pseudomonas* species bacteremia caused by contaminated normal human serum albumin. J Infect Dis 135:729–735, 1977

588. Stein PD, Folkens AT, Hruska KA: *Saccharomyces* fungemia. Chest 58:173–175, 1970

589. Steinhauer BW, et al: The *Klebsiella-Enterobacter-Serratia* division: clinical and epidemiological characteristics. Ann Intern Med 65:1180–1194, 1966

590. Stickler GB, et al: Diffuse glomerulonephritis associated with infected ventriculoatrial shunt. N Engl J Med 279:1077–1082, 1968

591. Stickler DJ, Thomas B: Sensitivity of Providence to antiseptics and disinfectants. J Clin Pathol 29:815–823, 1976

592. Strauch B, Andrews L, Siegel N, Miller G: Oropharyngeal excretion of Epstein-Barr virus by renal transplant recipients and other patients treated with immunosuppressive drugs. Lancet 1:234–237, 1974

593. Sumaya CV: Endogenous reactivation of Epstein-Barr virus infections. J Infect Dis 135:374–379, 1977

594. Sutnick AI, et al: Australia antigen (a hepatitis-associated antigen) in leukemia. J Natl Cancer Inst 44:1241–1249, 1970

596. Suwansirikul S, Rao N, Dowling JN, Ho, M: Primary and secondary cytomegalovirus infection: clinical manifestations after renal transplantation. Arch Intern Med 137:1026–1029, 1977

597. Swender PT, Shott RJ, Williams ML: A community and intensive care nursery outbreak of coxsackievirus B5 meningitis. Am J Dis Child 127:42–45, 1974

598. Talbot HW Jr, Parisi JT: Phage typing of *Staphylococcus epidermidis*. J Clin Microbiol 3:519–523, 1976

599. Taschdjian CL, Seelig MS, Kozinn PJ: Serological diagnosis of candidal infections. Crit Rev Clin Lab Sci 4:19–59, 1973

600. Telatar H, Kayhan B, Kes S, Karacadag S: HB Ag in sweat. Lancet 2:461, 1974

601. Teres D: ICU-acquired pneumonia due to *Flavobacterium meningosepticum*. JAMA 228:732, 1974

602. Teres D, et al: Sources of *Pseudomonas aeruginosa* infection in a respiratory/surgical intensive-therapy unit. Lancet 1:415–417, 1973

603. Terman JW, Alford RH, Bryant RE: Hospital-acquired *Klebsiella* bacteremia. Am J Med Sci 264:191–196, 1972

604. Thacker SB, et al: An outbreak in 1965 of severe respiratory illness caused by the Legionnaires' disease bacterium. J Infect Dis 138:512–519, 1978

605. Theologides A, Osterberg K, Kennedy BJ: Cerebral toxoplasmosis in multiple myeloma. Ann Intern Med 64:1071–1074, 1966

606. Thom AR, Cole AP, Watrasiew CZK: *Pseudomonas aeruginosa* infection in a neonatal nursery, possibly transmitted by a breast-milk pump. Lancet 1:560–561, 1970

607. Thomas M, et al: Hospital outbreak of *Clostridium perfringens* food-poisoning. Lancet 1:1046–1048, 1973

608. Thompson TR, Swanson RE, Wiesner PJ: Gonococcal ophthalmia neonatorum. Relationship of time of infection to relevant control measures. JAMA 228:186–188, 1974

609. Tiku ML, et al: Distribution and characteristics of hepatitis B surface antigen in body fluids of institutionalized children and adults. J Infect Dis 134:342–347, 1976

610. Tillotson JR, Lerner AM: Characteristics of pneumonias caused by *Escherichia coli*. N Engl J Med 277:115–122, 1967

611. Toivanen P, Toivanen A, Olkkonen L, Aantaa S: Hospital outbreak of *Yersinia enterocolitica* infection. Lancet 1:801–803, 1973

612. Tolkoff-Rubin NE, et al: Cytomegalovirus infection in dialysis patients and personnel. Ann Intern Med 89:625–628, 1978

613. Traub WH, et al: Characterization of an unusual strain of *Proteus rettgeri* associated with an outbreak of nosocomial urinary-tract infections. Appl Microbiol 22:278–283, 1971

614. Tuazon CU, Perez A, Kishba T, Sheagren JN: *Staphylococcus aureus* among insulin-injecting diabetic patients. An increased carrier rate. JAMA 231:1272, 1975

615. Tully JG, et al: Septicemia due to *Mycoplasma hominis* type I. N Engl J Med 273:648–650, 1965

616. Tully JG, Smith LG: Postpartum septicemia with *Mycoplasma hominis*. JAMA 204:827–828, 1968

617. Turbeville DF, Heath RE Jr, Bowen FW, Killam AP: Complication of fetal scalp electrodes: a case report. Am J Obstet Gynecol 122:530–531, 1975

618. Turck M, et al: Studies on the epidemiology of *Escherichia coli*, 1960–1968. J Infect Dis 120:13–16, 1969

619. Turkel SB, Overturf GD: Vaccinia necrosum complicating immunoblastic sarcoma. Cancer 40:226–233, 1977

620. Turner RA, MacDonald RN, Cooper BA: Transmission of infectious mononucleosis by transfusion of pre-illness plasma. Ann Intern Med 77:751–753, 1972

621. Uman SJ, Johnson CE, Beirne GJ, Kunin CM: *Pseudomonas aeruginosa* bacteremia in a dialysis unit. 1. Recognition of cases, epidemiologic studies and attempts at control. Am J Med 62:667–671, 1977

622. Valdivieso M, et al: Fungemia due to *Torulopsis glabrata* in the compromised host. Cancer 38:1750–1756, 1976

623. Valenton MJ, Brubaker RF, Allen HF: *Staphylococcus epidermidis (albus)* endophthalmitis. Report of two cases after cataract extraction. Arch Ophthalmol 89:94–96, 1973

624. Valman HB, Wilmers MJ: Use of antibiotics in acute gastroenteritis among infants in hospital. Lancet 1:1122–1123, 1969

625. Vandepitte J, Debois J: *Pseudomonas putrefaciens* as a cause of bacteremia in humans. J Clin Microbiol 7:70–72, 1978

626. Van der Wiel-Korstanje JAA, Winkler KC: The faecal flora in ulcerative colitis. J Med Microbiol 8:491–501, 1975

627. Vietzke WM, Gelderman AH, Grimley PM, Valsamis MP: Toxoplasmosis complicating malignancy. Experience at the National Cancer Institute. Cancer 21:816-827, 1968

628. Villarejos VM, et al: Role of saliva, urine and feces in the transmission of Type B hepatitis. N Engl J Med 291:1375-1378, 1974

629. Vogel L, et al: Infections due to gentamicin-resistant *Staphylococcus aureus* strain in a nursery for neonatal infants. Antimicrob Agents Chemother 13:466-472, 1978

630. von Graevenitz A, Mench AH: The genus *Aeromonas* in human bacteriology: Report of 30 cases and review of the literature. N Engl J Med 278:245-249, 1968

631. Wachsmuth IK, Stamm WE, McGowan JE Jr: Prevalence of toxigenic and invasive strains of *Escherichia coli* in a hospital population. J Infect Dis 132:601-603, 1975

632. Wagnild JP, et al: *Pseudomonas aeruginosa* bacteremia in a dialysis unit. II. Relationship of reuse coils. Am J Med 62:672-676, 1977

633. Wald ER, Synder MJ, Gutberlet RL: Group B β-hemolytic streptococcal colonization—acquisition, persistence and effect of umbilical cord treatment with triple dye. Am J Dis Child 131:178-180, 1977

634. Walzer PD, et al: *Pneumocystis carinii* in the United States. Epidemiologic, diagnostic and clinical features. Ann Intern Med 80:83-93, 1974

635. Wands JR, et al: Hepatitis B in an oncology unit. N Engl J Med 291:1371-1375, 1974

636. Ward R, Borchert P, Wright A, Kline E: Hepatitis B antigen in saliva and mouth washings. Lancet 2:726-727, 1972

637. Washington JA II: *Aeromonas hydrophila* in clinical bacteriologic specimens. Ann Intern Med 76:611-614, 1972

638. Washington JA II: The microbiology of evacuated blood collection tubes. Ann Intern Med 86:186-188, 1977

639. Washington JA II, Birk RJ, Ritts RE Jr: Bacteriologic and epidemiologic characteristics of *Enterobacter hafniae* and *Enterobacter liquefaciens*. J Infect Dis 124:379-386, 1971

640. Washington JA II, et al: Nosocomially acquired bacteriuria due to *Proteus rettgeri* and *Providencia stuartii*. Am J Clin Pathol 60:836-838, 1973

641. Weil AJ, Ramchand S, Arias ME: Nosocomial infection with *Klebsiella* type 25. N Engl J Med 275:17-22, 1966

642. Watanakunakorn C, Carleton J, Goldberg LM, Hamburger M: *Candida* endocarditis surrounding a Starr-Edwards prosthetic valve. Arch Intern Med 121:243–245, 1968

643. Weiner M, Werthamer S: *Corynebacterium aquaticum* septicemia. Characterization of the microorganisms. Am J Clin Pathol 64:378–381, 1975

644. Weinstein RJ, Johnson EH, Moellering RC Jr: *Candida* ophthalmitis—a complication of candidemia. Arch Intern Med 132:749–752, 1973

645. Weis J, Seeliger HPR: Incidence of *Listeria monocytogenes* in nature. Appl Microbiol 30:29–32, 1975

646. Weller TH: The cytomegaloviruses: ubiquitous agents with protean clinical manifestations. N Engl J Med 285:267–274, 1971

647. Wells GM, Woodward TE, Fiset P, Hornick RB: Rocky Mountain spotted fever caused by blood transfusion. JAMA 239:2763–2765, 1978

648. Welshimer HJ, Donker-Voet J: *Listeria monocytogenes* in nature. Appl Microbiol 21:516–519, 1971

649. Werder EA, Sonnabend W: Neonatal infection with *Streptomyces pelletieri*. Am J Dis Child 125:439–441, 1973

650. Wetli CV, Heal AV, Miale JB: A previously unrecognized laboratory hazard: Hepatitis B antigen-positive control and diagnostic sera. Am J Clin Pathol 59:684–687, 1973

651. Wheeler CE Jr, Huffines WD: Primary disseminated herpes simplex of the newborn. JAMA 191:455–460, 1965

652. Whitby JL, Blair JN, Rampling A: Cross-infection with *Serratia marcescens* in an intensive-therapy unit. Lancet 2:127–128, 1972

653. Whiteley GR, et al: Nosocomial urinary tract infections caused by two O-serotypes of *Providencia stuartii* in one hospital. J Clin Microbiol 6:551–554, 1977

654. Whiteside JD, Begent RHJ: Toxoplasma encephalitis complicating Hodgkin's disease. J Clin Pathol 28:443–445, 1975

655. Wilfert JN, Barrett FF, Kass EH: Bacteremia due to *Serratia marcescens*. N Engl J Med 279:286–289, 1968

656. Wilkinson HW: Analysis of group B streptococcal types associated with disease in human infants and adults. J Clin Microbiol 7:176–179, 1978

657. Wilkinson HW, Facklam RR, Wortham EC: Distribution of serological type of group B streptococci isolated from a variety of clinical material over a five-year period (with special reference to neonatal sepsis and meningitis). Infect Immun 8:228–235, 1973

212   Hospital–Associated Infections

658. Williams DN, Lund ME, Blazevic DJ: Significance of urinary isolates of coagulase-negative *Micrococcaceae*. J Clin Microbiol 3:556–559, 1976

659. Williams JW, Rittenberry A, Dillard R, Allen RG: Liver abscess in newborn—complication of umbilical vein catheterization. Am J Dis Child 125:111–113, 1973

660. Williams REO, et al: Nasal staphylococci and sepsis in hospital patients. Br Med J 2:658, 1959

661. Williams RJ, Govan JRW: Pyocine typing of mucoid strains of *Pseudomonas aeruginosa* isolated from children with cystic fibrosis. J Med Microbiol 6:409–412, 1973

662. Williams SV, et al: Epidemic viral hepatitis, type B, in hospital personnel. Am J Med 57:904–911, 1974

663. Wilson JF, Marsa GW, Johnson RE: Herpes zoster in Hodgkin's disease: clinical, histologic and immunologic correlations. Cancer 29:461–465, 1972

664. Winkhaus-Schindl I, Seeliger HPR, Andries L: Listeriose als gesicherte Ursache bei einigen Patientinnen mit habituellen Aborten. Geburtshilfe Frauenheilkd 25:1028, 1965

665. Winston DJ, Balsley GE, Rhodes J, Linne SR: Disseminated *Trichosporon capitatum* infection in an immunosuppressed host. Arch Intern Med 137:1192–1195, 1977

666. Winterbauer RH, Kraemer KG: The infectious complications of sarcoidosis. Arch Intern Med 136:1356–1362, 1976

667. Wynne JW, Armstrong D: Clostridial septicemia. Cancer 29:215–221, 1972

668. Young LS, Armstrong D: *Pseudomonas aeruginosa* infections. Crit Rev Clin Lab Sci 3:291–347, 1972

669. Young LS, Armstrong D, Blevins A, Lieberman P: *Nocardia asteroides* infection complicating neoplastic disease. Am J Med 50:356–367, 1971

670. Young NA, et al: Disseminated infection by *Fusarium moniliforme* during treatment for malignant lymphoma. J Clin Microbiol 7:589–594, 1978

671. Young RC, et al: Aspergillosis: the spectrum of the disease in 98 patients. Medicine 49:147–173, 1970

672. Zabransky RJ, et al: *Klebsiella*, *Enterobacter*, and *Serratia*: biochemical differentiation and susceptibility to ampicillin and three cephalosporin derivatives. Appl Microbiol 18:198–203, 1969

673. Zierdt CH, Williams RL: Serotyping of *Pseudomonas aeruginosa* isolates from patients with cystic fibrosis of the pancreas. J Clin Microbiol 1:521–526, 1975

674. Zinner SH, Daly AK, McCormack WM: Isolation of *Eikenella corrodens* in a general hospital. Appl Microbiol 25:705–708, 1973

675. Zinner SH, Garrity FL, McCormack WA: *Eikenella corrodens* and other similar bacteria: A review of laboratory aspects and clinical significance. Crit Rev Clin Lab Sci 5:193–200, 1974

ADDITIONAL GENERAL REFERENCES

Allen JC (ed): Infection and the Compromised Host. Baltimore: Williams & Wilkins Co., 1976

Altemeier WA, Culbertson WR, Hummel RP: Surgical considerations of endogenous infections—sources, types, and methods of control. Surg Clin North Am 48:227–240, 1968

American Hospital Association: Infection Control in the Hospital, 3rd ed. Chicago: American Hospital Association, 1974

Cundy KR, Ball W (eds): Infection Control in Health Care Facilities. Baltimore: University Park Press, 1977

James RD, McLeod CM: Induction of staphylococcal infections in mice with small inocula introduced on sutures. Br J Exp Pathol 42:266–277, 1961

Kunin CM, Edelman R (eds): The impact of infections on medical care in the United States. Ann Intern Med 89 (suppl):737–866, 1978

Mudd S (ed): Infectious Agents and Host Reactions. Philadelphia: W.B. Saunders Co., 1970

Polk HD Jr, Stone HH (eds): Hospital-Acquired Infection in Surgery. Baltimore: University Park Press, 1977

Proceedings of the International Conference on Nosocomial Infections—Center for Disease Control, August 3-6, 1970. Chicago: American Hospital Association, 1971

Roberts RB (ed): Infections and Sterilization Problems. International Anesthesiology Clinic, Vol. 10, No. 2. Boston: Little, Brown and Co., 1972

Samuels TM, Swidler HJ, Hawkins PA: Infection Control in Hospitals: An Annotated Bibliography. St. Paul: The 3M Company, 1975

INDEX